THE CULTURAL CONTEXT
OF HEALTH,
ILLNESS, AND MEDICINE

THE CULTURAL CONTEXT OF HEALTH, ILLNESS, AND MEDICINE

Martha O. Loustaunau and Elisa J. Sobo

BERGIN & GARVEY
Westport, Connecticut • London

Library of Congress Cataloging-in-Publication Data

Loustaunau, Martha O., 1938–
    The cultural context of health, illness, and medicine / Martha O.
  Loustaunau, Elisa J. Sobo.
      p. cm.
    Includes bibliographical references and index.
    ISBN 0–89789–487–1 (alk. paper). — ISBN 0–89789–548–7 (pbk.)
    1. Medical anthropology. 2. Social medicine. I. Sobo, Elisa
  Janine, 1963– . II. Title.
  GN296.L68 1997
  306.4'61—dc21   97–16136

British Library Cataloguing in Publication Data is available.

Library of Congress Catalog Card Number: 97–16136
ISBN: 0–89789–487–1
      0–89789–548–7 (pbk.)

First published in 1997

Bergin & Garvey, 88 Post Road West, Westport, CT 06881
An imprint of Greenwood Publishing Group, Inc.

Printed in the United States of America

The paper used in this book complies with the
Permanent Paper Standard issued by the National
Information Standards Organization (Z39.48–1984).

10 9 8 7 6 5 4 3 2

Copyright Acknowledgments

Grateful acknowledgment is given for permission to reprint from the following
sources:

Caring for Patients from Different Cultures by Geri-Ann Galanti. Copyright ©
1991 by the University of Pennsylvania Press. Reprinted with permission.

Walkin' Over Medicine by Loudell F. Snow. Boulder, CO: Westview Press, 1993.
Reprinted with permission of the author.

Contents

Abbreviations

AIDS	Acquired Immune Deficiency Syndrome
AMA	American Medical Association
CDC	Centers for Disease Control and Prevention
CMs	Complimentary medical practitioners
FAS	Fetal alcohol syndrome
HBM	Health belief model
HIV	Human Immunodeficiency Virus
IV	Intravenous
LBW	Low birth weight
NIH	National Institutes of Health
PO	Participant observation
PWHA	Person (or People) living with HIV/AIDS
SES	Socioeconomic status
SIDS	Sudden Infant Death Syndrome
STD	Sexually transmitted disease
WHO	World Health Organization

Introduction

People in all cultures confront illness, disability, and death: everyone gets sick, many become disabled, and ultimately everyone dies. Systems of health care exist within every culture, as a cultural universal. The ways in which we perceive and interpret health and illness, and seek and deliver care, are inextricably bound up with cultural norms, beliefs, and values, as well as with social structure and environmental conditions. This book focuses on the various dimensions of these relationships.

Previous treatments of health, illness, and medicine generally have not examined them together within a multicultural context. We feel that there is much need for such an approach, particularly in view of the increasingly multicultural character of the U.S. population. This approach not only reveals various relationships between social and cultural factors, but also points to many areas for fruitful social scientific research. Separate disciplines are often too narrow in their focus and interpretations; the use of cross-disciplinary viewpoints offers a broader, more illuminating perspective.

The subdisciplines of medical sociology and medical anthropology address health, illness, and medicine from very similar, sometimes overlapping, and yet often distinctive perspectives. Each discipline has its specific focus, terminology, and methodology, although there has been much cross-disciplinary borrowing. This text draws on the strengths of each discipline.

A BRIEF DISCIPLINARY HISTORY

Long traditions of research on medically related topics exist in both anthropology and sociology. But the formal subdisciplines of medical sociology and medical anthropology only began to emerge at midcentury.

Medical Anthropology

After World War II, medical anthropology (still at that time an unnamed specialization) received impetus and support from applied work in the arena of international public health. Good (1994) refers to the field in the 1960s as a "practice discipline," dedicated to the service of improving public health in societies in economically poor nations.

Despite the fact that this recent involvement with public health was key to its formal emergence, medical anthropology has old roots. These extend in two directions, reflecting two kinds of anthropology: biological or physical, and sociocultural. And while some anthropologists from both camps followed the public health line when it came along, some kept their interests purely theoretical. In any case, most medical anthropologists take somewhat of a systems approach, considering health and medical care within the context of cultural systems (Foster 1978).

Among biological medical anthropologists, major areas of study include biocultural phenomena such as diet, nutrition, and evolutionary adaptation. In the sociocultural branch of anthropology, which is the branch this book draws upon most, there has been a long-standing ethnographic interest in medical practices, knowledge, and beliefs as part of the total culture of peoples studied (Foster 1978: 3). Many socioculturally oriented theorists have recently turned toward analysis of illness representations and explanatory models, both in medical knowledge and popular social views of the body and of diseases, such as AIDS (e.g., Good 1994; Martin 1994). Social variables have been increasingly factored in as the links between sociology and anthropology have been strengthened (e.g., Augé and Herzlich 1995). Medical anthropology, however, has just begun to find its way into medical school curricula.

Medical Sociology

Medical sociology's history is quite different; the subdiscipline was situated within the framework of the scientific medical model, reflecting positivist values, viewing illness as a form of deviance (e.g., Parsons 1951). Changes in morbidity and mortality after World War II, the rise of preventive medicine, the establishment of modern psychiatry, and administrative needs contributed to medical sociology's rise (Coe 1978). Medical sociologists gained acceptance and credibility through applied work from within the medical field, finding faculty positions in medical schools. There was, however, little or no recognition that "medicine" includes diverse systems, all of which are influenced by the cultural contexts in which they are actualized (Gerhardt 1989).

While sociologists still focus on the dominant medical systems in both Europe and America, since the early 1980s the areas of interest in medical sociology, influenced by theoretical perspectives of social constructionism and the poststructuralist movement as well as growing popularity of critiques of medicine by Michel Foucault (see Foucault 1976 [1963]), have widened. They essentially cover four broad categories: (1) the relationship between environment and health and illness, (2) health and illness behaviors, (3) the relationship of health care practitioners with their patients, and (4) the health care system or the organization of health care delivery (Weiss and Lonnquist 1994: 6). Further, the variable of culture has become more significant in medical sociology; many researchers now consider biomedicine as a product of culture, as well as a culture in itself (e.g., Good 1994; Payer 1989).

A CHOICE OF TERMS

Much research in medical sociology and anthropology originates from within the perspective of European and American scientifically based medicine. This system is generally referred to as the "true" or benchmark medical system. In comparison, other medical systems, from Chinese acupuncture to Caribbean bush medicine, are often dismissed and devalued without consideration or understanding of possible functions or benefits. The dominant medical system is thus often referred to as *modern medicine, cosmopolitan medicine, Western medicine, clinical medicine*, or *biomedicine*. However, other medicines are practiced in this modern day, in cosmopolitan areas, in the West, in clinics, and with biology in mind.

In this text, we have chosen to use the term "biomedicine" when discussing the dominant medical system, since "bio" suggests that health and wellness are physiological issues, which are the focus of the medical model. We do note that other medicines may also be biologically grounded (albeit perhaps in biologies that differ from the mainstream version). We will also refer to our anthropological and sociological subdisciplines as "medical," since professional associations in the United States use the label, and with the understanding that the subjects covered go far beyond the generic term of identification.

"Science" is a term that can also be problematic. Many medical systems claim "scientific" systematized knowledge derived from observation and study. However, our use of science in relation to medicine refers to the series of systematic, organized steps that ensures maximum objectivity as well as consistency in research. This system, known as the scientific method, has produced discoveries and inventions from antibiotics and surgical success to genetic engineering and space travel.

Another terminological problem with which we have had to come to grips involves the national focus of the text. While it is true that much of what we say has implications for other economically developed nations, including most Western European nations, most of the research we cite in relation to biomedicine is written from a U.S. perspective. So, the generalizations that can be made from this work notwithstanding, when we refer to "our" society, we are referring to the United States. We use the term "America" to refer to the United States advisedly: America really is the name of a continent group, and there are many nations in the Americas.

One last problem with terminology involves the distinctions among the definitions of illness, sickness, and disease. While "disease" refers to the medical or pathological source of a problem, "illness" generally refers to the individual experience of being ill.

Sociologists use the word "sickness" for describing a social response to unwellness as a form of deviance. Unwellness requires a person to take on, at least temporarily, a social role, referring to societal expectations about the attitudes and behavior of the "sick" person. In anthropological jargon, the term "sickness" is used to draw attention to the social-structural causes of unwellness.

In any case, illness and sickness are often used interchangeably. We have attempted to use them appropriately, but recognize that meanings may become blurred and have therefore often used the term "illness" as a general designation.

THE SOCIOCULTURAL APPROACH: A CHOICE BLEND

George Foster, in his discussion of the disciplines of sociology and anthropology, noted the value of combining them in order to learn more by providing a broader perspective: "Precisely because we ask different questions, seek out different data, and come to conclusions that reflect our professional biases, our total understanding of medical and health phenomena is richer and more varied than if the task were left to a single discipline. We are in complementary, and not competitive, lines of work. We learn from each other, and we teach each other. Our society needs both of us" (1978: 10–11). As a sociologist (Loustaunau) and an anthropologist (Sobo), we agree.

Therefore, the basic focus of this text is to examine the role of cultural differences in defining and dealing with health and illness and to investigate the health-related factors that link humanity cross-culturally through common needs, using our two related disciplines. Each perspective gives us specific knowledge and understanding of the many elements that make up health and illness behaviors and systems. Both perspectives recognize how an appreciation for and an understanding of cultural diversity, as well as commonalities, are essential for developing a unified and effective system of health care delivery in our distinctly multicultural nation.

The United States encompasses a great variety of ideas, philosophies, and practices within a core system for delivery of health care to a diverse population. This core system is based upon a biomedical model that generally has not supported cultural awareness and sensitivity in health care delivery, recovery, or rehabilitation. It has also given little recognition to alternative healing systems and beliefs that exist side by side with biomedicine and that are often used instead of or in conjunction with mainstream care.

The U.S. population grows increasingly culturally diverse. Drawing from the knowledge of both sociology and anthropology, we examine how our cultural backgrounds, our diverse beliefs and values, and our societal structures are related to our physical and mental health. What are the various ways people perceive health and illness, and how do those perceptions affect related behaviors? What political and economic issues are involved? How and why does the health system that is meant to care for all of us incorporate or exclude those cultural aspects of our identities that play such a large part in our health status? How can we improve this system's ability to provide the best possible quality of life for those it serves?

THE TEXT: A PREVIEW

In Chapter 1, we examine the concept of culture and establish its significance with relation to health and illness. The role of culture is explored in terms of personal identity and behavior and its consequent links to health, disease, and illness.

Issues of ethnocentrism, cultural relativism, and multiculturalism are addressed in relation to social and political controversy, and the difficulties of finding a balance between diversity and unity are explored. We suggest that medical care that excludes diverse cultural factors and considerations falls short of addressing human needs that must be met.

Chapter 2 explores the influence of social structure and related variables in causes of and approaches to health and illness in our multicultural society. The pivotal roles of kinship and family, ethnicity, social class, and gender are shown to shape how both consumers and providers perceive and deal with illness and maintain health. These variables are also examined as sources for and causes of illness and of discrimination in and barriers to care-seeking and treatment.

The different stages of our lives entail different health and illness challenges and require different approaches to care and coping. Chapter 3 addresses birth and childhood, adolescence, adulthood, and old age; it investigates the many and diverse cultural issues associated with these life stages. Issues of sexuality, maternal-child health, and death are also discussed in relation to cultural context, focusing on their implications for health care on the personal and structural levels.

All cultures have socially sanctioned as well as limited, marginalized, quasi, and auxiliary modalities of treatment. Chapter 4 defines and discusses a number of these modalities. It includes an examination of intercultural differences and commonalities and ways in which many of these modalities may be complementary. Dangerous therapies and quackery are also discussed as they relate to cultural relativity, individual choice, and legal concerns. We stress the need for education of both providers and consumers.

Chapter 5 takes a look at the United States as a multicultural nation and examines how the health care system evolved from its diverse folk roots into the now-dominant biomedical culture. Various cultural contributions and institutional values, as well as technological developments and the emergence of powerful political and economic interests, have all played roles in the formation of the American health care system and the resulting dominance of the biomedical system.

Biomedicine is characterized as both a part of the larger culture, reflecting its mainstream norms, values, and beliefs, and as a culture in itself, based on the classical scientific model, with its own language, structure, norms, values, and beliefs. Biomedical culture is also viewed in terms of various elements, including service versus profit orientations in care delivery, changing patient- or client-practitioner relationships, the process of medicalization, ethical concerns as they are fueled by increasing costs and exploding developments in technology, and the increasing recognition of the limitations of the biomedical paradigm for addressing emerging social and medical problems.

Methods for gathering and assessing cultural information are the focus of Chapter 6. This chapter centers on problems of cross-cultural communication. Besides language differences, problems of cultural relativity, error and misunderstanding, and ethnocentrism all must be overcome. This chapter suggests various methods that may be utilized by practitioners and caregivers in order to more effectively serve culturally diverse populations.

We tie the lessons of previous chapters together in Chapter 7, which illustrates the approach we recommend as it discusses the connections between AIDS and culture. Since cultural attitudes, perceptions, beliefs, and norms are very important in the transmission of HIV, they are, therefore, equally important in the educational approaches to AIDS prevention.

This chapter also suggests how the various modalities and themes addressed throughout the text might be combined and integrated to provide more sensitive, effective, humane, and accessible health care. The need for cooperation and inclusion rather than narrowly focused and competitive models is stressed. Issues of cost, power, relativism and diversity, communication, and respect for human rights must be considered with the aim of moving toward a more realistic model of health care delivery in an increasingly pluralistic world.

Goals and Considerations

This book was not written to answer all of the very difficult questions raised by the challenging problems of health care delivery in a multicultural society. It does, however, emphasize the links that have been identified between sociocultural systems and the health and well-being of a population. What those links are, and their role in the provision of just and humane health care, is a main focus of this volume. Biomedical concepts and contributions are not denied, but the present system of biomedicine cannot be considered outside of a cultural context. Rather, biomedicine must be seen to be a part of the social environment and, therefore, as subject to and as influenced by culture as every other system.

From a multicultural perspective, our primary question is how to retain and utilize a knowledge of and respect for cultural diversity in care delivery while maintaining a sense of unity in the face of common difficulties of suffering across cultures. Inclusion of an understanding and appreciation of cultural diversity and commonality in the education of health care providers, as well as of patients, is vital and essential for creating a system that effectively cares for all citizens.

In covering the topics included in this text, we have had to be selective. In-depth discussions of all relevant culturally related issues would require many books. The best we can do here is to provide an overview. To this end, we have tried to include ideas and research from numerous perspectives within our respective disciplines and thought-provoking discussions on current (often controversial) issues. Our purpose is to generate in the reader the motivation and capability to recognize and understand culturally related factors that influence our views and constructions of health, illness, and healing, as well as of science and medicine.

Our project was not one that we could carry out alone. While we, alone, are responsible for this work, shortcomings and all, we are indebted to our colleagues for their insightful and critical comments and suggestions, and for kindly permitting us to quote from their works. While we do not have the space to name all who contributed, those to whom we owe thanks include Helen Ball, Fred Bloom, Robert Echenberg, S. Malia Fullerton, Geri-Ann Galanti, H. Jack Geiger, Kate Hill, Pat Hippo, Jill Kerr, Tamara Kohn, Terry Meyer, Mark Nathan, Milagros Pena, Billy Reeves, Andrew Russell, Charles Sanders, Robert Simpson, Loudell Snow, Adina Sobo, and Wenda Trevathan, not to mention our long-suffering spouses, Joaquin Loustaunau and Harvey Smallman.

For future efforts, we welcome comments, criticisms, suggestions, and case examples from all readers.

1

The Concept of Culture

If anything was made to be taken for granted, it is culture.
[Gallagher and Subedi 1995: 4]

Goal: To explain and analyze the concept of culture and identify its components and elements through anthropological and sociological approaches.

Goal: To examine ethnocentrism, cultural relativism, and multiculturalism and to become aware of their meanings, controversies, impacts, and significance for health care in the twenty-first century.

Culture is present in all aspects of life. And yet, until faced with a contrasting culture that challenges the basis of our beliefs, values, and identity, we generally do take our own culture for granted. In the area of health care provision, cultural diversity and the experience of contrasts is increasing. This affects the relationships of patients and providers and the outcomes of their interactions, as well as the relationships between and among providers themselves. In an increasingly multicultural society, it thus becomes essential for effective and humane health care that all of us learn more about culture—to understand what it is, how it functions, and its relevance for our interactions and their outcomes.

WHAT IS CULTURE?

In attempting to understand and analyze health and illness in any society, individual behaviors, interactions, and social structures must be placed within a cultural context. A **culture** is, put briefly, all the shared, learned knowledge that people in a society hold. A **society** generally consists of people who share a specific geographical area within which they interact together, guided by their culture.

Culture guides how people live, what they generally believe and value, how they communicate, and what are their habits, customs, and tastes. It guides the ways people meet the various needs of society: how goods and services are produced and distributed, how power and decision-making are designated, what god or gods are represented (if any). Culture prescribes rituals, art forms, entertainment, and customs of daily living. Most certainly, the ways in which we interpret and perceive health and illness and our choices in providing and seeking care are influenced by our culture.

Culture is a kind of knowledge that we use and act on. Some of this knowledge is declarative in that it consists of apparently factual information ("Mint tea is good for digestion."). Some of it is procedural, or how-to, information ("Boil a handful of mint leaves in water until the water turns dark; pour this water into a cup through a strainer and drink when cool enough."). Cultural knowledge of both kinds exists in relation to all realms of existence, including subsistence or food production, economics, kinship, government or the maintenance of order, religion, gender, leisure, and health and illness. Importantly, cultural knowledge can be changed or adapted by its users to fit new conditions. A group's culture is always evolving as the life circumstances of the group change (see Wedenoja and Sobo 1997).

Dominant Cultures and Subcultures

The United States is considered to be a **pluralistic** society in which multiple cultures ideally exist side by side in harmony. Basic institutions are also shared by all, including the political, economic, and legal systems as well as a common language. Pluralism as an ideal, however, is greatly endangered by prejudice, discrimination, and selective immigration policies. Pluralism is also qualified. Where multiple cultures mix or meet, as they do in the United States, the society must promote some sense of consensus among all members concerning basic norms, ideals, beliefs, and values. The mainstream or **dominant** culture (sometimes referred to as a **core** culture) is the one whose norms, values, language, structures, and institutions tend to predominate.

In the United States, the dominant culture has typically been white due to colonization by people of Western European origins. Williams (1970) identified fifteen of what he considered to be major themes and orientations representative of the dominant culture in the United States, which for the most part are relevant today:

1. Personal achievement and success

2. Hard work and productivity

3. Humanitarianism and support of the "underdog"

4. Orientation toward moral judgments of events and situations

5. Pragmatism, or practicality and efficiency

6. Progress toward a better life

7. Materialism and consumerism

8. Equality for all

9. Freedom and individual autonomy

10. Outward conformity, as in dress, recreation, housing, and political expression

11. Science as a tool of mastery over the environment

12. Nationalism and loyalty to that which is "American"

13. Democratic principles and belief in everyone having a voice in political matters

14. Individual importance and responsibility

15. Racism and the idea of group superiority

Some of those themes indicate conflicting values such as the value of equality (the idea that all people have a right to health care) and an emphasis on racism and related group superiority (which results in denial of care to those without insurance or who cannot pay—generally members of various disadvantaged racial and ethnic groups and, most recently, illegal immigrants).

Contradictions like these are common in all cultures. Cultural changes, such as those produced by the civil rights movement of the 1960s, often come about in the ongoing attempt to resolve the contradictions in core orientations. Such changes may bring about new contradictions and may even produce a backlash.

Another result may be the formation of deviant cultures, or **countercultures**; these entail alternative lifestyles for those who cannot conform to or actively oppose widely accepted social norms. Since biomedicine is considered a part of the dominant culture in the United States, those alternative medical movements that reject the biomedical approach, such as Christian Science, exist, at least in terms of medical systems, as countercultures.

While countercultures emerge in opposition to the dominant culture, a **subculture** is generally considered a group within a larger group: a subgroup (meaning a subset, with no implication of inferiority) that lives within the general norms of a dominant group while preserving, to an extent, the roots and lifestyles unique to them. The differences between cultures and subcultures may be based on political affiliations, socialization experiences, language, ethnicity, age, religion, occupation, health status such as disability, class, or gender.

The various health care professions also form subcultures. When a person decides to become a doctor, for example, s/he will learn not only a new vocabulary, but will also acquire a way of seeing that goes with that vocabulary. As a Harvard medical student explains, " 'In a sense we are learning a whole new world . . . because learning new names for things is to learn new things about them. If you know the name of every tree you look at trees differently. Otherwise they're just trees' " (Good and Good 1993: 98).

Regarding patients, another student said, " 'At first you are very aware that you are dealing with another person. Now I just don't think about that any more. You just do the routine' " (Good and Good 1993: 101). Adds another, " 'I've had some real perception changes of people. . . . More and more, I can't help but think of us as machines' " (96). Becoming a doctor—or an acupuncturist, or nurse, or Vodun (sometimes spelled Voodoo) priestess, or any kind of health worker—is a process of acculturation as much as the result of long hours of hard work and study.

Subcultural groups and their members may be **bicultural**, functioning equally within their traditional milieu and the dominant culture; traditional, holding to their own traditions while rejecting many of the dominant ones; **marginal**, having little to do with either cultural group; or **acculturated**, having given up most of the traits of their original cultures and adopted those of the dominant group (Locke 1992: 6). Various groups may have become acculturated to a greater degree in some areas than in others. For example, they may reject the biomedical explanation of disease and its modes of treatment while fully accepting the dietary habits and patterns of dress of the dominant culture.

The United States is full of acculturating—and acculturated—people. However, **enculturation** (cultural socialization from birth) is such a powerful process that health crises often lead even the most highly acculturated people to return to their original cultural patterns (Galanti 1991: 112). Seriously sick or injured people may also return to their native language and require a translator when brought in for care. It is therefore extremely important that the health provider have an appreciation of the various cultures and cultural nuances of the people s/he serves.

Is Culture All?

Despite the foregoing, behavior is not determined solely by culture, nor any other one factor. A mental framework holding that one force determines how we think and behave is called determinism. Environmental determinism thus posits that we are as we are due to the climate or environment of the geographic area we inhabit. Biological determinism holds that biology or genetic factors are key.

Biological factors surely do play a role in determining some dimensions of human lifeways. Genetic research, for example, is revealing various information about one's odds of contracting various inherited diseases. However, some biological determinism is in actuality thinly disguised racism.

The case of erroneous arguments that I.Q. (a measure of intelligence) is determined by race is an example of such. Biased findings indicating that Whites are intellectually superior to other groups are used to justify white oppression of nonwhites as biologically determined, or natural. But cross-cultural data show that the intelligence measured by I.Q. testing is shaped by class and culture, not by race (see Fraser 1995).

This is easily seen in data from a study of children's intelligence carried out a quarter of a century ago. The study (Cole 1975, as cited in Nunley 1995) tested children's grasp of the idea of conservation, "the idea that when you pour all the water from a short glass into a tall glass, the same amount of water is still present, or if you take a fat ball of clay and roll it into a long narrow string of clay, the same amount of clay is there" (Nunley 1995: 76). The study was carried out with children of potters in Mexico and children in a West African fishing village. When water was used, the fishing village children did better, but when clay was used, they were outscored by the potters' children.

The majority of research shows that racial differences in I.Q. mask inequalities linked to poverty and limited life chances. Further, differences have little significance in terms of actual intelligence, in that they measure only a narrow (and culturally determined) type of cognitive achievement (Gross 1992: 222–23).

In the **nature versus nurture** debate, nature, or biology, is pitted against nurture, or culture, as the explanation for the human condition. In reality, neither is true; both positions are too extreme and too simplistic. Real human thought and action is the outcome of a complex interplay of cultural, biological, social, psychological, economic, and political variables. However, in anthropology as well as in sociology, culture is indeed quite key.

ETHNOCENTRICITY, MEDICOCENTRICITY, AND CULTURAL RELATIVISM

Culture Blindness

Culture from either the anthropological or sociological perspective can be seen as a measure of human flexibility. Its study reveals the amazing diversity of ways and means of meeting human needs under all sorts of conditions. It is both an abstraction and a blueprint or guide for social analysis. By studying the various elements of culture we can begin to understand different social groups, the cultural contexts in which they function, and the links between cultural context, healing institutions, and human behavior related to illness and help-seeking.

Loudell Snow has worked for over twenty years on the topic of African American medical practices. Snow describes the case of John and Eva Thompson (pseudonyms). The Thompsons had brought their baby Patty to the pediatrics clinic for her first immunization. Snow, affiliated with the clinic in her capacity as an anthropologist, sat in on the consultation (1993: 95).

The doctor administered the shot and then asked if there were any questions, and the parents had none. However, as soon as the doctor left the room, Mrs. Thompson turned to Snow and asked if she had ever heard of using catnip tea for colic. As Snow tells it, "I replied that I knew it was a popular remedy in the neighborhood—but that I had always wondered how people knew how strong to make it. Mrs. Thompson's response was, 'Why it *says* right on the box!' " Mrs. Thompson also told Snow that adding a bit of honey made the tea taste better to the infant, and she and her husband told Snow a few other things about their medical traditions as well as their medical history—things that the attending physician should have been told (1993: 95–96; italics in original).

When Snow shared with the physician the important medical history information that the woman and her husband had provided, she was annoyed. " 'I don't know why these people always tell *you* everything' " (1993: 96; Snow's italics), she said to Snow. "It does seem obvious," Snow reflects, "that the initial question about catnip tea was a test: Mrs. Thompson clearly knew about catnip tea for colic, exactly how to prepare it, and, in fact, was already using it. Had I responded in a negative fashion she probably would not have gone on" (97). The Thompsons were worried about the possibility of being negatively judged for their practices—of being the victims of ethnocentrism.

Ethnocentricism involves using one's own standards, values, and beliefs to make judgments about someone else. The standards against which others are measured are understood to be superior, true, or morally correct, while those being evaluated and not "measuring up" are inferior or wrong. Ethnocentrism can be observed in all types of cultural, social, and even personal evaluations when we condemn the customs, ideas, behavior, values, and beliefs of someone else when they are different from our own.

Ethnocentrism can also be observed regarding the tenets of science and medicine, which as noted may be considered natural or "correct" and therefore outside of cultural considerations. This attitude has been termed "medicocentrism" (Pfifferling 1981: 197). A **medicocentric** view focuses on disease, identified through signs and symptoms, and not on the patient or the patient's perception of a problem. The medicocentric physician uses a **reductionist** model, trying to make a diagnosis by narrowing (or reducing) the problem to medically explained phenomena (**disease**). But the patient may attempt to expand and relate the problem to his or her own perceptions and experiences, such as an inability to carry out daily functions, symptom recognition and interpretation, misfortune, and discomfort (**illness**).

Physicians, as products of their own cultures, as well as of their medical training and occupational subculture, may exhibit both ethnocentric and medicocentric attitudes, which compound the problem of bias. Let us say, for example, that Ms. Jones, a working-class, divorced, black woman has come to see Dr. Smith, a white, Anglo male, who has confirmed her suspicion that she is pregnant. Dr. Smith also finds that she is malnourished and requires a great deal of prenatal care. He does not think that unmarried, working-class women should have babies. He lectures her on the use of birth control and pointedly mentions the option of sterilization. Medically, he prescribes diet, vitamins, and possibly medication, as well as time off work and some light exercise, without considering that Ms. Jones cannot afford the prescriptions or that she must continue working in order to pay the rent. The probability of her compliance is extremely low (see DiMatteo and DiNicola 1982, ch. 5).

Cultural Relativism

The concept of **cultural relativism** requires that we do not judge, but consider actions, beliefs, or traits within their own cultural contexts in order to better understand them. It involves maintaining a sense of objectivity and an appreciation for the values of other cultures. It asks what functions various cultural elements serve and how they are sustained, not whether they are "good" or "bad" by external standards. Cultural elements are deemed not better, not worse, just different.

Cultural relativism presents some difficulties, particularly in health care, in that some cultural beliefs and practices may be harmful or may be based on cultural biases that in turn may cause harm. They may even have legal implications from the perspective of the dominant culture.

One such culturally related belief and practice concerns female genital surgery, sometimes referred to as female genital mutilation, or FGM, which is practiced in a number of countries. The hood of the clitoris, the clitoris itself, or the clitoris as well as both the inner and outer labia are removed. The latter form of the operation, which is most common in the Sudan and Nubian Egypt, is called infibulation (D. Gordon 1991: 5). As Daniel Gordon explains, "the two sides of the wound [are] then stitched together, leaving a small pinhole opening for the drop by drop passage of urine and menstrual blood" (5).

The practice of FGM is based on an ideal image of the female body as lacking certain parts of or all external genitalia (as opposed to male bodies, on which external genitalia are expected), and the belief that by removal of these body parts females will not become sexually active or desirous and will remain virgins until marriage and will be faithful afterward. Moreover, the clitoris is considered "dirty," and the female is not fit for marriage until it has been removed and she is "clean" (D. Gordon 1991: 9). One folk name for female genital operations is **tahara**, or purity. FGM, based solely upon cultural values and interpretations, is excruciatingly painful, nontherapeutic, and medically can be very dangerous (Toubia 1994).

Novelist Alice Walker, an activist against the practice, fought attempts to legalize FGM in the Netherlands as an "expression of culture" for those immigrants who engaged in the practice (Walker and Parmar 1993). FGM has also been observed in the United States in immigrants from the Arab and African countries where the custom is most widely practiced, and some immigrant groups are said to be importing specialists to perform the ritual. Physicians in the United States who have seen the results of FGM have strongly condemned it. As reported in the *New England Journal of Medicine*, "Female circumcision, or female genital mutilation, can no longer be seen as a traditional custom. It has become a problem of modern society in Africa as well as in Western countries. In recent years, concern has grown over how to stop the practice, rather than whether it is appropriate to intervene" (Toubia 1994: 716).

Intercultural contact produces diffusion, adaptation, innovation, and change, hopefully for the better. Cultural relativism in relation to human rights can easily be defended on the basis of the fact that all cultures are in constant flux; that is, even so-called tradition changes and, therefore, traditional practices need not be cast as sacrosanct. Traditions may become outmoded and impractical. But all people have certain rights by virtue of being human. Although idealistic, this stance is encoded in the International Bill of Human Rights (United Nations 1978). Furthermore, as acts of torture, terrorism, oppression, persecution, poverty, suffering, and disease in any society have repercussions around the globe, they cannot be viewed from a culturally relative perspective.

HUMAN SIMILARITY, HUMAN DIVERSITY: THE MULTICULTURAL SOCIETY

The health care system increasingly treats individuals from multicultural backgrounds, and by its very nature, the system should not be selective in who is given care and treatment. The idea of care implies attention to all individuals and not just to a physical ailment. That includes respect for cultural identity.

The questions of cultural diversity go far beyond the institution of medicine, however, and engage the entire society. Arthur M. Schlesinger Jr. (1992) finds that "The question America confronts as a pluralistic society is how to vindicate cherished cultures and traditions without breaking the

bonds of cohesion—common ideals, common political institutions, common language, common culture, common fate—that hold the republic together" (Schlesinger 1992: 138).

The perceived threat of multiculturalism concerns fears of divisiveness,
the loss of traditional mainstream values, and interracial and ethnic hostility. The values and promises of equality that produced the rising demand
in the 1960s for equal opportunities and respect, as well as pride in diversity, produced a backlash against racism and discrimination and brought
some numerous and long overdue changes. The core culture, however, has
too often diverged from these values and promises, and we are now witnessing a backlash against diversity, as evidenced in the rise of hate crimes,
slurs, jokes, and public statements denigrating various minority groups, in
calls for legislation to make English the official language, and in the roll-
back of civil rights legislation.

Nevertheless, many of our core values are values to which all cultural
groups can relate, such as opportunities for a better life for one's children
(Glazer 1994). The uniquely American creed includes common ideals of
dignity, equality, inalienable rights, freedom, justice, and opportunity for
all human beings (Myrdal 1944). The fact remains that the United States
is and always has been a multicultural society, and demographic predictions
are that "multiculturalization" will continue and increase (U.S. Bureau of
the Census 1993b).

In the case of health and medical care, the ethnocentric and medicocentric orientations are justified as based within the scientific paradigm and,
therefore, with some possible exceptions, as not subject to a multicultural
or even a cultural analysis or cultural considerations. However, as we shall
see, in medicine, too, there is a need for both cultural knowledge and consideration, as well as for finding the balance between the meaning of our
cultural differences and those commonalities that unite us all.

CULTURE, HEALTH, AND ILLNESS

Culture affects our perceptions and experiences of health and illness in
many ways, and these perceptions and experiences change as culture
changes. Health problems of any group can be affected by a multitude of
cultural variables, some very basic. How we learn to subsist may depend
upon the available foodstuffs and our abilities to adapt and utilize our
environment. Custom and habit may produce sanitary or unsanitary living
conditions. For example, the diets of migratory hunter-gatherer people were
dependent upon the environment and climate. Because they moved from
place to place, they never stayed around one area long enough for their
own waste to bring about health problems.

The rise of agriculture, and then urbanization, created all manner of environmental health hazards in poor sanitation, overcrowding, starvation, and new vectors or conduits for disease. Technology has solved some of these problems primarily in developed countries, and then created others, including pollution, more lethal weaponry, and toxic chemicals.

Other cultural variables are more conceptual. For instance, we have different ideas about health itself. A sociological study in France (Pierret 1995 [1983]) identified four ways of defining what health is: people saw health as either (1) the absence of illness, (2) a resource, (3) a controllable product of the individual, or (4) a "collective heritage for which society is responsible" (195). These understandings seemed to be linked to social class or to people's position within a society.

What is illness to one person, or one culture, may be no problem to another, and vice versa. For example, in some cultures, what we in the United States call mental illness is not only *not* classified as illness, but is interpreted as favor from God in allowing an individual to understand or see what others cannot. Among the Navajo, for whom the prevalence of congenital hip disease is relatively high, treatment is simply not seen as necessary. Although it can eventually be painful, the condition is not seen as significant; resultant limping carries no stigma for the Navajo, while it does for the mainstream American (Adair, Deuschle, and Barnett 1988: 206–7).

Ideas about the visible signs of health also differ; for example, many mainstream U.S. women strive for thinness, while in impoverished Jamaica, a plump female body is much more appealing (Sobo 1994). The people of Fiji also like fat bodies, as these signify a wealth of social connections and financial resources and, thus, "health" (A. Becker 1994).

Cultures also differ on ideas of treatment for common health problems and on preventive measures. To keep fit, a white American might go for a daily walk or join a health club to work out, while an African American might, in addition or as an alternate, take a laxative purge in the spring and several other times throughout the year (Snow 1993). A Native American might attend a "sweat lodge" ceremony in order to purify and renew the spirit (Kunitz 1983).

Health problems can be attributed to pathogens, accidents, or physical degeneration; they also can be attributed to supernatural means or relationships that do not meet idealized cultural standards, and they may be treated accordingly. In many cultures, health problems index social problems, as we will see. And they can entail not only physical symptoms, but behavioral or emotional problems as well.

The subsequent chapters contain many examples of cultural influence in all areas of illness, disease, sickness, and healing. In the next chapter, we look more closely at the role of specific cultural and institutional structures that influence the ways we interpret health and illness, as well as the ways we care for ourselves and others who are sick.

FOR DISCUSSION

1. In what way are you a member of a culture or subculture? Identify some of the customs that characterize the groups to which you belong.

2. Discuss some instances in which cultural relativism might or might not be appropriate. Identify some instances of ethnocentrism that you have witnessed or heard about. What are some examples of ethnocentrism in health care?

3. What are the major issues in the debate over multiculturalism, and what are ways in which those issues relate to health care?

2

The Health-Related Consequences of Social Structure

Much of the tension in the clinical encounter ... does not derive from the existence of diverse health subcultures, nor is it due to a failure in medical education to instill an appreciation of folk models of health and illness; rather, it is a reproduction of larger class, racial, and gender conflicts in the broader society.

[Singer 1995: 85]

Goal: To understand how the social structure influences our positions and interactions with regard to our health, illness, and care-seeking and delivery.

Goal: To appreciate the related significance of the specific structural elements of family, ethnicity, social class, and gender in our health, illness, and care-seeking and delivery.

All interactions take place within complex social settings. Focus on beliefs and behavior (as expressed in healer-patient relationships), definitions and perceptions of health and illness, and decisions on whether or not to seek care and from whom has too often resulted in a neglect of the sociostructural factors that influence those behaviors and interactions (Clark, Potter, and McKinlay 1991).

While we may be interested to know how healers make their diagnoses or how people in different cultures decide whether they are well or ill (topics we examine in chapter 4), knowing cultural rules is not enough. A consideration of social structure can tell us a great deal more about why people act the way they do.

Just as each society has a culture or cultures to guide its members, each society also has a **social structure**. This refers to the organized patterns of relationships between individuals and groups within a society, which orders their behavior in a predictable fashion and influences their interactions. Like culture, social structure can be seen as a social construction, that is, the product of social and power relations that have complex histories and are not fixed, but are subject to change.

Cultural beliefs and notions support, call for, explain, and sometimes even mystify or mask structural arrangements involving kin, class, and gender, so that such arrangements are perpetuated. For example, the cultural value that health care should be available to every citizen may mask the reality that the structure of medical care delivery is not set up for such provision. If the system is not seen as requiring change, efforts to change it will most likely fail.

Similarly, social, political, and economic structures support and make essential certain cultural ideals or forms. Laws concerning the acceptable form and structure of the family, for example, support cultural norms concerning marriage (e.g., that it be monogamous and that it occur between a man and a woman who are not closely related). In this chapter, we begin to explore the interdependence between social structure and cultural expectations by examining concepts of family, ethnicity, gender, and social class.

THE FAMILY: A CULTURAL UNIVERSAL

All societies are divided in some way along the lines of **kinship,** which defines who is related to whom and in what way. Rules of descent and family structure will vary from group to group according to various cultural patterns. Further, the importance of kinship also will differ. But all individuals belong to kindreds or families, whether they know these families or not.

Everyone who descends from the same line of ancestors belongs to the same **lineage.** In a unilineal system, a person is related by blood only to one parent's lineage. For example, the Navajo are **matrilineal** (Adair, Deuschle, and Barnett 1988: 249). Therefore, a Navajo child belongs only to her mother's lineage. She is not related to her father's siblings' children as cousins in the same way as a British or American girl would be. Those cousins are members of a different lineage. Ideas about relatedness have implications for medical record-keeping and affect people's notions of what runs in the family.

Domestic Units

The domestic group most typically referred to by the term "family" in the United States is the **nuclear family,** which consists of a married mother (female) and father (male) and their unmarried children, living together. The marriage is considered monogamous and is, according to the ideal, sanctioned by U.S. law, which prohibits more than one spouse at a time.

A **blended family** is formed when couples previously married with children get divorced and remarried, and then have more children together. There are also single-parent families, childless families, and gay families where the couple are of the same sex. The **extended family** consists of one of the above family units plus one or more grandparents, or may include an offspring's children, aunts and uncles, or other relatives.

Although nuclear, blended and extended family units all, ideally, center around **conjugal** pairs (one male and one female), many families entail no such couples. That families without conjugal pairs are seen as aberrant is reflected in the terminology used to describe them, such as the "broken home" or even "dysfunctional" family. These terms imply that there is something wrong with a family in which there is a single parent. But single-parent families are only aberrant from the vantage point of a culture that idealizes a dual parenting arrangement and certain restrictive sexual arrangements. While in the United States the nuclear form is seen as the preferred family arrangement, only approximately one-fourth of households fit this model (U.S. Bureau of the Census 1990: 2).

A household generally involves a group of people who share living space at a given point in time, and who usually are—but need not be—kin. One person can also constitute a household. Household members sleep in the same complex and generally share food. A household is essentially an economic unit; it jointly produces goods or pools money and purchases commodities like power, water, and food.

People may belong to more than one household. In the United States, disadvantaged children's clinic records often contain multiple addresses, identify several different household heads, and list several different last names for members of any one household. Children may spend the day with one household and sleep in another (Snow 1993). Household members change as different friends and relatives come and go in response to the changing events in their lives, representing a strategy for survival under harsh circumstances (Stack 1974).

Fictive Kin

A common American cultural variation of the family involves **fictive kin**, or people who are talked about and treated like kin with the full knowledge that they are not *really* related. Fictive kin may take responsibility for such things as protection, education, and health care of people who are not truly kin to them. Such flexibility is often seen among Blacks and people of Caribbean heritage. Urban black children with multiple caretakers tend to be less fearful about and friendlier toward strangers than their white counterparts, who seem to suffer more separation anxiety as a result of a rigid caretaking ideal in which a child can have only one mother figure (Snow 1993: 234).

Sometimes, fictive kinship entails ritual action and formal behavioral specifications. For example, many people of Mexican heritage (and Roman Catholics of other origins) practice *compadrazgo*, or godparenthood: parents invite men and women to act as co-parents when a child is expected and then born. The godparents are responsible for helping out, adopting, or fostering the child should anything happen to the parents. Pediatricians and clinicians working with populations that practice *compadrazgo* should be aware that sometimes they will need to deal with up to four co-parents of one little patient, or that a culturally legitimate (if not legally sanctioned) adoption has taken place.

Family can be more usefully defined by function rather than structure; the family's functions, like structures, may vary, but are generally related to support, whether moral, emotional, physical, financial, social, or psychological. Functions may include protection, socialization, regulation of sexual behavior, affection and companionship, and provision of social status. They may also include reproduction, which contributes to human survival, or material, economic production, which also has benefits for survival. An often forgotten but essential function is the delivery of health care (Pratt 1976: 2).

In Sickness and in Health

In many societies, the household or family delivers much of the health care. It is what has been referred to as the "hidden health care system" (Freund and McGuire 1995: 174). The family functions as a support system and as a cost containment mechanism when, as a unit, its function has been disrupted by the illness or dysfunction of one or more members.

Even in a large-scale complex society, the patient who seeks health care is not afflicted solely as an individual. Rather, s/he is affected as part of a family unit, and the entire group may be affected by his or her ill health. So, treating the patient also involves treating the family. Knowledge about various patterns of family structures and the need for family involvement is, therefore, essential for effective health care delivery in a multicultural society.

In biomedicine, the links between households and ill individuals are minimized, and treatment centers on the individual body. However, some biomedical professionals now recognize that what happens in the household does affect and is affected by an individual's sickness. In a broad review of biomedical literature on family-centered health care, David Schmidt (1978) cites a number of studies demonstrating a positive correlation between poor health outcomes and the level of stress in a home (as measured by such things as unemployment, communication problems, having a member with a chronic illness, a recent experience of divorce, death, or desertion, etc.). For example, in one study high household stress correlated with a steady increase in streptococcal acquisition, illness, and a rise in antibodies (305). High stress also was related to increased risk of stroke (305), angina or chest pain (307), and concern with one's own and one's children's **somatic** (physical) symptoms (309–10). Pregnant women with high stress and low levels of social support had a pregnancy complication rate of over 90 percent (305).

Schmidt also found that when one's spouse has a disease, one's own somatic symptoms are quite likely to increase. And certain chronic diseases appear in both spouses at a rate that is significantly higher than might be explained by chance (1978: 309). There were links between spousal death and the death of the remaining spouse from a number of causes, including tuberculosis, hypertensive heart disease, influenza, and pneumonia (306). Likewise, divorce can be unhealthy because of the stress it entails in certain contexts. Where divorce is not condoned, or when only one party seeks it, stress is heightened (see also Holmes and Rahe 1967 for relationship of stress and illness).

It has also been found that good communication between clinicians and family members, and good family relations, correlates with good rehabilitative progress (Schmidt 1978). Compliance with clinician's recommendations also is better among clients with support from family members. For example, family empathy and support was shown to increase compliance in alcoholism treatment, to hasten the recovery process in stroke victims, and to elicit good response in patients with severe orthopedic disabilities.

On the basis of his review, Schmidt argues that there is "a definite advantage" in taking the family as the unit of medical care (1978: 303). Thus, in patient diagnoses, health care providers should be aware of the possible effects of life events, particularly those related to the whole family, and make appropriate referrals for treatment.

Women's Contribution to Health Care

Family care, notes Debbie Ward, a nursing professor, implies that all members of the family are involved in the caring, when they are not. "Family" is a code word for "women," used when discussing care at home (1993: 20).

Despite ideals of gender equality, in the United States women are still seen as nurturing caregivers and therefore are held responsible for health-related household tasks. Women bear the principle burden of care delivery for injuries or acute illnesses with sudden onsets, as well as for the chronic and long-term problems of disabled and elderly family members (D. Ward 1993). The burden falls most heavily on low-income women, often ethnic minorities, who have surviving traditions of large families and of caring for their disabled and elderly.

The **household production of health** involves more than just curing and caring; it also entails the daily round of cleaning, cooking, and child-minding activities. Women also bear the main burden of these jobs, often working a double day, both outside and inside the home; their own health can suffer accordingly (D. Ward 1993). Exploitation of families—and especially of women—as bearing the entire burden may create further problems of stress and impoverishment.

Family involvement in care of family members, however, can also help offset the problem of rising health costs. For example, family members can be taught to give injections, monitor diets, and help with other forms of therapy in order to avoid costly hospitalization (Schmidt 1978).

Many people have the idea that home care is free, saving the rest of society a heavy financial burden. But this does not take into account wages lost by those who temporarily leave the work force, losses in opportunity for job promotions and pension benefits, and the cost in the health and well-being of the caregiver, who then may become unwell and poor and must in turn rely on kin for unpaid care (D. Ward 1993). Additional costs involve various sacrifices the family as a whole must make in terms of its own financial needs, including saving for children's education and parents' retirement. However, much more research is needed on the actual burdens and consequences of care-giving.

Care and the Changing Family

In the past, without technology to keep us alive for longer periods of time and under more severe circumstances, the length of time spent caring for disabled or frail elderly family members was limited. Further, changes in family structure wrought by industrialization have produced difficulties. First, the size of the average household has declined, mostly due to a rise in single-person and single-parent households (Chadwick and Heaton 1992). Female-headed households increased from 21.1 percent to 28 percent of total households from 1970 to 1989, while single male-headed households rose from 8.3 to 15.9 percent in the same time period. For Blacks and Hispanics, female-headed households comprise over 40 and 23.1 percent of total households, respectively (Chadwick and Heaton 1992).

One family in six is now headed by a single woman, and more than one-third of female-headed households are poor (Naisbitt and Aburdene 1990: 46). Besides the decrease in husbands' support for wives, other changes in family structure include cohabitation, dual career or employment patterns, fewer children, and the fact that more children are living with someone other than both parents. Estimates suggest that many people are involved in the care of other family members to the limits of their abilities. Cultural assessment may become an especially useful tool for medical care providers in determining the burdens and abilities of individual families to be a part of caregiving while remaining a viable family unit that can function socially and financially.

A Growing Health Hazard: Domestic Violence

A growing family health problem is domestic violence, which produces physical, mental, and emotional damage and is generally (but not always) carried out against women and children. Domestic violence is not a new problem, but it is one that has been kept hidden within the family itself, covered up with bogus explanations, like stories of accidental falls, when seeking medical care (Gayford 1994).

Only since the 1970s has public disclosure revealed a terrible and extensive picture of violence within an institution meant to nurture and protect. Given the cultural values of family autonomy, health professionals may still look for easy answers or ignore the problem. They may also feel helpless in the face of the reality of violence within the domestic sphere and fall back on the claim that their role is to heal visible wounds, not to intervene in situations beyond their expertise.

Many factors are involved in domestic violence, including alcohol and drug use, psychiatric disorders, personality problems, jealousy, and various types of stress, social isolation, lack of coping skills, and social learning (Gayford 1994). Once taught to recognize the signs of domestic violence, health care professionals are in a good position, if trust of the victim can be gained, to recommend counseling, psychological treatment, and in extreme cases, referral to a shelter (in the case of children, many states have laws requiring reporting of suspected violence). But the major weapon against domestic violence would seem to be a change in social values. Health care professionals can promote the idea that domestic violence is no one's right, is not acceptable, and should not have to be tolerated.

Providing Care for the Family

Problems of costs and care are not being addressed either politically, economically, or medically. A number of possible solutions to the general problem of family care for the disabled, elderly, or chronically ill are simply not considered on any broad scale because they do not fit within the cultural constructs of the society with regard to families and care. Some solutions, suggested by D. Ward (1993: 24–25), include superior adult day-care centers; new types of housing designed for different types of families; institutionally based care in the home, with families providing some assistance; community and public service centers combining health clinics;

day care for elders and preschool children; community lunch facilities; housing partnerships; and shared spaces like apartments linked to community health workers' offices, and services for cleaning and meal preparations. Such possibilities will continue to face strong opposition as long as society assumes that the problem of chronic care is the responsibility of, and will be addressed by, families (mostly women—and some men) and that such care is free and has no cost to the society or to individuals.

Perhaps the message for all caregivers, both professional and lay, is to take time to understand the power and limitations of the family, whatever the culture and however structured, in health, illness, and recovery or in simply maximizing quality of life for everyone concerned. Family structure and environment are essential elements in a patient's diagnosis, treatment, recovery, or rehabilitation.

Fuller and Toon (1988), in discussing the various family structures related to minority populations, include two propositions for dealing with families with a structure different from that of the practitioner. First, there is the need for at least an intellectual understanding of any given family structure and its dynamic—how it functions. Second, there must be an emotional acceptance that different types of family structure may operate with the same degree of success (or failure) as the structure accepted in the practitioner's own culture (69).

Families are composed of different kinship ties and relationships, but they are still families with strengths and problems. Some families have more resources than others, some have strong beliefs relating to health, illness, and caregiving, but all are subject to general social and economic conditions that affect abilities to respond to health and illness, whatever the cultural or ethnic origin.

The concept of family covers a broad range of structures and functions and may be defined slightly differently according to ethnicity, social class, and gender. Like family structures, ethnic, class, and gender identities also affect and influence the perceptions, relationships, and responses of both health care givers and receivers, as well as the general structure of caregiving institutions. They are also linked into the global political economic system, such that habits—and health problems—that seem to be local or individual may actually have been engendered by larger sociopolitical considerations.

THE CONCEPT OF ETHNICITY

Ethnicity is tied to notions of shared origins and shared culture. In the United States, ethnicity is reflected in the classifications of Mexican American, German American, and Polish American, for example. Even without an explicit national or continental qualifier, all Americans are members of one or another ethnic group. White, middle-class, American ethnicity, for example, can be identified through commonly preferred television shows, modes of dress, and viewpoints, including views on who qualifies as a member of their group.

Ethnic groups form when one group of people assumes an identity different from those with whom they share borders. These borders can be national boundaries, but they also can be based on the distribution of power in a society and factors on which this power is based, such as skin color, religion, language, and country of origin.

The ethnicity "Native American" emerged when America was colonized. Aspects of the divergent identities of the many existing tribes merged when groups who previously might have been enemies came together in a united effort to resist colonization and cultural annihilation.

Ethnic identities are constantly being invented and modified. Further, they are not necessarily permanently fixed to the individual, although they may be ascribed on the basis of visual criteria. Skin color cannot be easily changed, but its cultural significance can vary. And specific practices entailed in an ethnicity can be forgotten or adopted not only by whole groups but also by individuals (such as in giving oneself a new name or in forgetting one's native language). In this way people can, under certain circumstances, merge with or separate from a specific ethnic group.

An individual may have many ethnic identities, especially in a multicultural setting. And these can, in certain situations, be used selectively: individuals can shift back and forth between identities as they see fit. For example, a clinician or client may use English in the clinic setting and another language at home. One may eat certain foods when lunching with colleagues at work or in a clinic waiting room, but may eat different foods at home. Adopting a role specific to another ethnic group does not imply hypocrisy; as different contexts call forth different dimensions of the self, a person may simply be exhibiting the self that is most pertinent in a given situation (Goffman 1959). Or, of course, one can be playing the system in an effort to "pass," to get by, or to avoid problems such as being discriminated against, subjected to harassment, physical violence, or even killed.

Minority Status and Health

Members of certain groups may have very little input into the social system that governs them. This **minority** status reflects their lack of opportunity, access, and participation, rather than number. Minority status, in turn, affects health status.

For example, like other migrant workers, Mexican migrant workers travel continually as crops are ready for harvest. Their health care is fragmented, with no follow-up or continuity. Further, migrants usually work through the heat of the day with little or no time to rest or cool off. Employers sometimes fail to supply accessible toilet facilities, and with open fields and no shelter, people sometimes wait the entire day to urinate or defecate, creating various intestinal and kidney ailments. Water is sometimes not supplied for hand washing, and so, after picking crops dusted with insecticide, workers ingest toxic substances with their lunches (see R. Baer 1996 and Bollini 1995). Before they were outlawed during the 1980s, short-handled hoes were used for harvesting, causing workers to stoop over for extended periods of time in the fields, creating spinal and associated problems.

Black Americans have also, as a group, suffered poorer health than white Americans. As Ernest Quimby notes, "Poor health is a structural feature of Black existence" (1992: 161). In other words, poverty, powerlessness, and the racism that these conditions are tied to, severely limits the health care options open to Blacks, while greatly expanding their health challenges (see Lazarus 1990; M. Ward 1993a). For example, infant mortality rates are twice as high for Blacks as for Whites—or more, depending on where data are collected. For instance, in Michigan the 1988 infant mortality rate for black babies was 21.9 per 1,000 live births, while for white babies it was 8.6 per 1,000 (Snow 1993: 172). And the infants that do survive are challenged in their fight for survival: a study of mortality rates carried out in New York City revealed that men in Bangladesh, an impoverished and underdeveloped nation, are more likely to reach the age of 65 than are black men in Harlem (McCord and Freeman 1990, as cited in Snow 1993).

Racism is pervasive in the health care system (see Funkhouser and Moser 1990). As Janis Hutchinson (1993) notes, it exhibits itself in cursory physical examinations, deficient bed assignments, delayed admissions, and assumptions of noncompliance; further, racism often overlaps with class-based discrimination against the poor, and it influences the adoption, implementation, and administration of health policies that limit certain aspects of the lives of lower-income people. As Hutchinson points out, "Access to health care in the USA is usually dependent on ability to pay for it" (1993: 10–11), and many Blacks are poor (U.S. Bureau of the Census 1993b). Navarro (1994) notes that the problems are rooted in the social structure, and that "it is unlikely that by concentrating solely on race differentials we will ever be able to understand why the health indicators of our minorities are getting worse" (494).

Self-Perceived Compliance versus Noncompliance

Mrs. Hibbert, an African American, was told by her doctor never to eat pork, so she gave it up. However, as Loudell Snow reports (1993: 142–43), Mrs. Hibbert never extended her understanding of pork to include pork fat. She served Snow a tasty lunch of greens and cornbread, prepared with liberal portions of bacon grease. Even as she cooked, she talked about her doctor's instructions and how much she missed ham.

In another case reported by Snow, a man diagnosed with high blood pressure stopped taking his pills. When he went in for his monthly exam, the staff was shocked to see that his pressure was elevated. They asked about his medication, and he freely admitted not taking it. He reminded the staff that a blood test he had been given last time indicated that he should stop the medication. This caused much confusion, for the only blood test the man had been given was a routine blood count. But then he reminded them that the doctor told him that his count was a little low. The man took this to mean that his blood pressure medication had thinned his blood out and needed to be discontinued until balance was restored (Snow 1993: 134).

Misunderstandings, such as those Snow reported, are responsible for a good deal of what clinicians patronizingly call "noncompliance." However, some clients do not want to take medicines prescribed and do not intend to do so. This is the case across the board, for all ethnic groups. Among the black population, this can be because clients see doctors' medicines as too strong, too chemical, or addictive (Snow 1993: 271). Many prefer their own home remedies to those that doctors might prescribe. They may go to the doctor for diagnoses, then, not for treatment. Others go simply to make sure that their own treatments are doing the job or that their health conditions are under control.

Ethnicity and Mistrust

Sometimes clients do not adhere to clinic recommendations, such as to take medications, because they fear being poisoned. In the United States, this is particularly so for people of African heritage. An elderly midwife explains:

You know a long time ago black people were treated so dirty and so they was afraid of doctors givin em a dose of somethin just because they was black. They had that in their mind. And from the way they were treated, they had a right to think of such. They . . . [say, "That doctor] may give me the black bottle["]. . . . Means poison. Something like that just to get rid of em. . . . [And people] thought the doctors would do some kinda experiment on em. Removin this and removin that cause it wasn't nothin but a black body. (Logan 1989 as quoted in Snow 1993: 266)

Many link black fears about the intentions of white health professionals directly to Blacks' knowledge of the historic and exploitive Tuskegee Syphilis Study. The study, which began in the prepenicillin year of 1932, involved documenting the natural course of untreated syphilis in about 400 poor black men. The men were manipulated into participating in the study with promises of free biomedical treatment and financial incentives.

The study was originally planned to be **cross-sectional**: it was to involve a single, time-limited effort in which researchers would examine men in various stages of syphilis to ascertain the damage that it would theoretically do over time to a (male) body. The original recruits did receive the then-standard heavy metals therapy (which involved mercury and arsenicals). But then authorities decided to turn the study into a long-term **longitudinal** effort, and cases were to be observed until "end point"; that is, until autopsy. The men did not receive antibiotic therapy when it became available in the 1940s (Edgar 1992; Jones 1992).

Exposure of the study by the media in 1972 led to its termination and, ultimately, to the passage of the National Research Act in 1974. The act mandated that proposals for all federally funded research involving human subjects be reviewed by boards that may reject any proposals deemed unethical or scientifically misguided.

In any case, the Tuskegee research—research funded by the U.S. government's Public Health Service—involved letting people die. Knowledge of this fuels rumors. For example, people often assume that the Tuskegee participants were intentionally infected with syphilis. While such assumptions may be false, the historic facts of the study cannot be denied. The feelings and knowledge that lead people who do hear about the Tuskegee study to draw erroneous conclusions often stem from life experiences. And, as James Jones points out, perceptions of racism and mistreatment are validated by the knowledge of the study's existence in a way that causes people who learn about it to cling to it as "a symbol of their mistreatment by the medical establishment, a metaphor for deceit, conspiracy, malpractice, and neglect, if not outright racial genocide" (1992: 38). The personal experience of racism as well as the legacy of the negative encounters that Blacks have had with the public health system fuel the misgivings that many minorities have about health care workers' motives and intents.

Some minority health problems do appear to be genetically linked, such as Tay-Sachs disease in Semitic peoples, sickle-cell anemia in Blacks, and diabetes in Native and Mexican Americans. African Americans, particularly women, also appear to be more prone to hypertension and diabetes (U.S. Department of Health and Human Services 1992: 31–39). However, the social structure contributes greatly to various susceptibilities and risks, as through poverty, and connections between stress and hypertension (Dressler 1990).

Ethnicity, Genetics, and Body Ideals

Genetically linked differences extend, to a certain degree, to visual characteristics such as skin color, facial features, and hair texture. While these traits will differ more according to one's specific genetic background than to one's purported race, members of minority groups have been known to be pressed into having plastic surgery so that their features are made more "mainstream."

Often, operations are justified as being beneficial to health. This is the case with upper eyelid surgery, by which some Asian people effect a more Anglo appearance. It can be rationalized as a biomedically necessary procedure to remove what some doctors call "excess fat" (Kaw 1993: 81) and to fix eyes that are "too narrow" (82). In other words, some doctors medicalize and cast as defective a quite natural facial feature. Eugenia Kaw reports that some women in her study were told by their doctors "that it was 'normal' for them to feel dissatisfied with the way they looked" (81). Unfortunately, this kind of racism is still all too common; clinicians today must work to correct it.

Minority peoples also have been made to feel bad about overall body shape and size or ways of styling the hair that do not conform with mainstream U.S. standards. For example, some African Americans who wear dreadlocks or beaded and braided hairstyles have been ordered by employers to alter their hairstyles. Hygiene concerns may be voiced to rationalize such orders, although dreadlocked or beaded braided hair is much less likely to be shed than is hair in a straight or loose white mainstream style. And people whose body ideal is plumper than the thin mainstream cultural ideal have been pressured to lose weight, even though we now know that the ideal weights used by insurance companies to indicate health risks change periodically and may be underestimated, and that some people are naturally heavier than (and just as healthy as) others. While obesity has generally been found to be unhealthy, the cultural perception, including that of biomedicine, of what constitutes obesity is variable (Mumford 1983: 148–49).

THE EFFECTS OF POVERTY AND SOCIAL CLASS

Socioeconomic Status

Conditions that may at first glance appear to be correlated with ethnicity or other variables may actually be due to relative poverty and, thus, to social class. **Social class** in the United States is generally measured by a combination of income, occupational prestige, and educational variables; together, these yield one's socioeconomic status (SES) and a general classification of upper-, middle-, or lower-class membership.

The United States is characterized as having an **open-class** system, which means that there is a great deal of social mobility between class categories or levels, and that social position is earned, or **achieved**. This structure is the opposite of a closed system, known as a **caste** system, where social position is **ascribed**, or assigned, at birth and in which there is no social mobility. In actuality, most systems—ours included—lie somewhere in-between. Various ascribed characteristics, such as ethnicity and gender, may also affect our opportunities for achieving higher social positions.

The dominant ideal cultural value of equal opportunity in the United States reflects the myth that "anyone can make it in this society if they really want to." Real values limiting social mobility through discrimination by ethnicity, sex, age, religion, and socioeconomic status are revealed in **structural barriers**. These barriers may consist of poor educational facilities and preparation, denial of employment in certain fields, of few or no promotions to positions of power, and of consistently low wages and lack of benefits for certain groups. Poor health or disability also can block social mobility.

Sickness and Poverty

Since poor people are definitely sicker than the well-off, largely because of poverty conditions, their **life chances** (meaning opportunities for acquiring favorable life experiences) are affected through loss of opportunities for advancement of personal and social goals (Gerth and Mills 1958). Barriers to mobility may also be created for family members who must care for those who are ill.

The ill or disabled may also be seen as lacking skills that they actually do possess, so they face discrimination much in the same way that members of ethnic minority groups are discriminated against. Much of poor health and disability is seen as a personal condition to be blamed on individual behavior. This ignores the role of social structure as a causal factor.

While poverty causes much sickness, in some cases it is true that sickness may cause poverty. For example, a person who becomes ill with a long-term catastrophic disease (AIDS, for example) may be denied both employment and insurance and may expend all his or her resources and savings to the poverty level. This theory of reverse causality is sometimes called the selective drift hypothesis. Although this idea may apply in some cases, it is not adequate to explain all cases. As a total explanation, it conveniently shifts the attribution and responsibility for poverty from the social structure to illness and the individual. With the exception of chronic mental illness, well-designed studies have failed to support the general contention (Hertzman, Frank, and Evans 1994: 77).

Ethnicity, Gender, and Financial Power

By any measure, ethnic minorities and women are at a distinct disadvantage regarding financial resources or control. A good part of this disadvantage can be attributed to structural factors such as the types of jobs available to these populations and the prevailing wage scales. As the hourly wage fails to respond to the cost of living, people find themselves working two or three jobs just to meet basic needs or perhaps not meeting them at all. Types of jobs held by this population include unskilled labor and service jobs that pay very little, offer few benefits, and are vulnerable to periodic layoffs.

Although risk factors are multiple and complex, studies consistently show higher rates of mortality, morbidity, and disability among the lower classes (see Pappas et al. 1993: 103–9). Explanations have included all the concomitants of poverty—poor housing, more exposure to pathogens, unemployment, poor education, less access to health care, discrimination, strenuous and dangerous working conditions, poor sanitation, and high stress. Additional factors would include higher risks for violence, high levels of drug and alcohol use, and high-risk sexual behaviors, which can also be related to social structural pressures.

Access and Utilization

Present patterns indicate that low-income groups became the highest utilizers of health care, with the most physician visits, after the institution of the national insurance programs of Medicaid and Medicare in the 1960s. They are followed by those in the middle income range, with the highest income group now having the lowest number of physician visits (Cockerham 1995: 120). This suggests that easier access increases usage, while more education and more preventive care lowers it.

Relative to need, the poor may still underutilize services. Although inadequate insurance coverage is a factor, so is a lack of emphasis on preventive care and denial of illness due to the more pressing needs of survival, such as the need for food and shelter. Poor people generally receive treatment for symptoms at home rather than preventive care and, thus, may be sicker when they do seek official medical help. In general, cultural perceptions and variations tend to be less important than economic necessity in the decision to seek care (Dutton 1978).

The factor that best explains low utilization in relation to need is what Dutton (1978) calls the "systems barrier." This involves location, availability of, and transportation to facilities and time needed for consultation and the negative experience of poor patient-physician or patient-provider relationships. The poor are also more likely to be uninsured or to receive Medicaid funds, which many doctors do not accept, so the places of treatment for the poor are more likely to be hospital outpatient clinics and emergency rooms. There, the patient is likely to spend more time in the waiting room, receive a lower quality of care or therapy, deal with more bureaucratic agencies, and be treated simply to return to the environment that may have contributed to poor health in the first place.

Access to biomedical care, however, still falls far short of explaining class differentials in health status and life expectancy: "persons in lower class groups have higher morbidity and mortality rates of almost every disease or illness, and these differentials have not diminished over time" (Syme and Berkman 1994: 29–35). Several studies done in Great Britain, where health care is more readily available to all through the National Health System, show that the provision of health care to poor populations did not affect the levels of disease and illness in that population; nor did it eliminate the difference in health status between social classes (Hollingsworth 1981; Reid 1989; Marmot, Shipley, and Rose 1984; Whitehead 1990). Patterns also emerge from U.S. data indicating that morbidity differentials by class are much larger than by race (NCHS 1988). Both Blacks and Whites in lower socioeconomic groups had higher rates of illness than Blacks and Whites at higher income levels.

Syme and Berkman (1994) point to the existence of gradients in which the lower the social class, the greater the mortality and morbidity rates. The differential includes virtually all disease conditions. They point out, "That so many different kinds of diseases are more frequent in lower class groupings directs attention to generalized susceptibility to disease and to generalized compromises of disease defense systems" (31). This suggests again the connection of mind-body, social conditions, coping mechanisms, and physical, psychological, and cultural vulnerability; it also suggests the need to focus on how the stress of poverty and discrimination may compromise the immune system making one more vulnerable as stress increases. Learning to cope may help alleviate stress, thereby lowering the risk of illness. However, there is a danger in focusing on individual coping and the idea that teaching people to cope with their poverty or life changes will solve the problem. Simply blaming people for not coping—or for coping through the use of tobacco, alcohol, narcotics or drugs, and violence—would relieve any pressure on the inequalities or responsibilities of the social system. And with no real change in the expanding structural environment of poverty, there will be no *real* change in the health of the poor. Personal responsibility, participation, and public education are necessary and vital, but poverty as part of the social structure must be addressed as an essential part of social change if we are to improve health status and quality of life for all in a permanent way.

For health care providers, an understanding and empathy for low-income patients and the effects of poverty can go a long way toward making such patients more comfortable and satisfied, opening up avenues for care-seeking and health education. It is also essential for those providing care to examine their own attitudes, beliefs, and motivations relating to racism.

Because there are so many variables that may be contributing to the patient's illness, it is vital to try to discern something more about their lives and environments than simply their SES classification (see chapter 6). It is also useful to have some knowledge of support systems, agencies, and contacts where some help may be found, including referral services, social workers, food supplement programs, support groups, or other public services and agencies.

Although we have emphasized poverty's effects on health and health-related behavior here, the effects of economic advantage should not be forgotten. They are implicit in statistics on the health of the poor. The health of those with economic means is the yardstick by which poverty's effects can be measured. Wealth confers power, and also affects attitudes toward health workers, as the following hospital case study shows.

The study further shows that the influence of social factors, such as class, rarely occur in isolation. The privilege that class buys the individual described below is augmented by the structure of gender relations that he draws on when dealing with the nurses assigned to him when he was treated in a hospital in his new country, America.

HAMID SADEGHI

*[Hamid Sadeghi] was a twenty-five-year-old upper-class Iranian. . . .
He was very uncooperative and refused to do anything for himself.
He would ring for the nurses and demand, "You get here right now
and do this." He would not, however, accept anything he had not
specifically requested, including lunch trays and medication. He
posted a sign on his door that read, "Do not enter without knocking,
including the nurses." His attitude caused a great deal of resentment
among the nurses. Why did he treat them this way?*

*When asked, Hamid responded, "This is the way it is done." Finally, one of the nurses who had an Iranian brother-in-law recognized
the behavior and explained. Traditionally, Iranian men are dominant
over Iranian women. They give orders to women, not take them.
Furthermore, as a member of the upper class, Hamid was probably
used to giving orders to servants. He was not purposely being difficult
but merely acting in his customary manner. (Galanti 1991: 23)*

Mr. Sadeghi's wealth gave him the upper hand in most of his social relations, and he expressed his power even in the hospital setting. The influence of wealth on his expressions of power toward female nurses was fortified by the structure of gender relations in his culture. In order to fully appreciate the culturally and socially constructed nature of the sway that such structures can have on health and health-related interactions, a deeper exploration of gender is called for.

GENDER ISSUES

Gender or Sex?

While **gender** differences have to do with ideas about what it is to be masculine or feminine, **sex** has to do with biological differences between males and females relating to reproductive functions. Sex differences are, for the most part, genetically determined. Babies are sexed according to the type of external genitalia they are born with.

This method of categorizing individuals generally works fairly well. But in some cases, internal biological signals become mixed or muddied, resulting, for example, in individuals who exhibit the external sexual characteristics of both sexes (Richardson 1988; Money 1980). Some are born internally male and externally female, or the reverse. The genitalia are not a foolproof indicator of genetic sex. Of course, the idea that one's genetic sex is somehow one's true sex is itself culture-bound. So are the ways in which male-female biological differences are perceived. Where biomedicine today sees differences between the male and female reproductive systems, other cultures' versions of biology see similarities. So even sex, which is a biological category, is not necessarily an unarguable natural fact.

Notwithstanding, the technical concept of sex differentiates us into male or female. Gender is manifest in socially and culturally constructed roles and expectations for behavior, along with a division of labor assigned to each gender, and present in all societies to one degree or another. Notions of gender, or of masculinity and femininity, generally entail the assumption that certain abilities, traits, and capacities fitted to particular tasks and activities are specific to each sex.

Gender is generally ascribed in a way that squares with perceived sex: males are generally brought up to act and think in a (culturally defined) masculine fashion, and females in a (culturally defined) feminine one. Gender socialization affects one's life chances as well as one's behavior and thoughts in that certain educational, occupational, and even health opportunities have often been reserved for one gender or the other.

Gender and Power

While many gender-linked associations are culturally specific, others are found cross-culturally and can be explained as based in fundamental differences between male and female physiology. For example, because of their biological childbearing role and because they can breastfeed, women cross-culturally are generally highly involved in caring for infants. Some theorists argue that it is precisely because women are so busy with childcare that men have been able to hold the power in many societies (e.g., Sacks 1974).

In such societies, which are called **patriarchal**, men are in control, and the more patriarchal a society is, the less important women and all that is associated with them are deemed. This devaluation serves an ideological function, supporting male domination. Negative stereotypes of women also may stem from what Bruno Bettelheim calls "procreation envy" (1962). In other words, men may feel jealous that women can have babies and they cannot. One way that men can gain the upper hand is by trivializing women's procreative power. So, for example, menstruation and birth become associated with nastiness and uncleanliness; menstruating women are banned from certain places or tasks. Further, sensibilities and skills associated with the female gender are devalued.

In addition to trivializing female functions, men may appropriate women's procreative power. They can do this in various ways. Bettelheim describes certain male-only religious rituals in which men perform sacrifices and other acts designed to ensure fecundity. If women's fertility depends on men's rituals, then men are the true masters of childbirth. Medicalization is another way by which men control women's procreative power, and we discuss this process in chapters 3 and 5.

Early European stereotypes of women as breeders and nurturers and men as property owners and controllers that were part of a patriarchal and patrilineal system of inheritance (Turner 1995) have survived in various forms in modern societies—even within the medical institutions. This is reflected in gynecological textbooks (Scully and Bart 1979) and in the occupational division of labor. Even in the face of contradictory evidence, old gender stereotypes remain strong, due to people's beliefs that gender roles are "natural" (biologically determined) or divinely ordained. Ultimately, the strength of these stereotypes may derive from political expediency in that they support vested interests in maintaining economic control of resources and the current distribution of power.

Nature or Nurture?

Anthropologist Margaret Mead (1935) described typical behaviors of each gender in three different cultures in New Guinea—the Mundugumor, the Arapesh, and the Tchambuli. When compared to American behavioral expectations for men and women, Mead found considerable differences.

In two of these cultures, there was little gender-role differentiation; one might say that these were one-gender cultures. Both male and female roles in the Arapesh were what would be considered feminine by U.S. standards—both were equally maternal, gentle, and home-loving. The Mundugumor would have been considered masculine—both males and females were hostile and fierce, seeming to care little for their children.

In the third culture, the Tchambuli, the role expectations were the reverse of those found in the United States. The women were solid, practical, and powerful providers who hunted and fished. The males were emotional, concerned with their appearance, enjoyed decorating their homes, and pursued the arts (Mead 1935).

If females are by definition indeed passive, overly emotional, nonintellectual, weak, submissive, and nurturing then all females in all societies should exhibit these characteristics. The same would be true for all males being stoic, rational, active, intellectual, and so on. Mead found that this was not the case. Biology, in other words, is not destiny.

Sexuality

Sex has to do with biology; gender, with culture; and **sexuality**, with the expression of erotic desire. In the United States and in similar cultures, two genders are all that are allowed. American ideas about gender include the assumption that to be masculine is to desire sex with women and to be feminine is to desire sex with men. These ideas, which are not universal cross-culturally (Davis and Whitten 1987: 81, 83), support the current American family-based norm of one mother (female) and one father (male) and are sanctioned by law and religion. Therefore, bisexual and homosexual identity and behavior (i.e., sexual attraction to and interaction with people of either sex or one's same sex, respectively) may be seen as not only nonnormative but as immoral and a threat to the entire society (Abelove 1994). Homosexual and bisexual people are thus subject to a great deal of hostility, stigma, and discrimination in the general society.

Alfred Kinsey's 1948 study of sexuality showed that in a population of 5,000 white American males, 37 percent reported at least one homosexual experience to orgasm as adults. This calls into question the definition of homosexuality in men. How many experiences—if any—must one have to be labeled homosexual? Many individuals who have repeated same-sex liaisons do not identify themselves as homosexual or gay and many who have no sex at all do identify as such. Further, many people who would be labeled, either by themselves or society, as homosexual actually frequently engage in heterosexual intercourse (Gatter 1995).

Homosexual behavior is practiced by people of all cultures and is found in all classes, occupations, and professions, including medicine. Because of oppression, many gay men and lesbians remain "in the closet," unwilling to allow their sexual orientations to become known.

Homosexual people face real barriers to quality health care because their sexual health needs are often ignored or denied. Health clinics rarely display posters or pamphlets depicting same-sex couples, but heterosexual pairs are frequently used. Women seeking pap smears or other regular gynecological screening may simply be assumed to be heterosexually active; questions such as "What type of birth control are you using?" can effectively stifle candid discussion of homosexuality (or asexuality or abstinence for that matter).

Moreover, at least for homosexual men, homophobia exacerbated by the AIDS pandemic has led to stigmatization and discrimination in health care settings. For those who do have AIDS, or the virus connected with it, the burden is double: some clinicians have refused to treat them. The American Medical Association (AMA) has decreed it unethical to refuse to treat pa-

tients with HIV/AIDS (see Stine 1993: 363–64). If general safety procedures, such as using surgical gloves and properly disposing of body effluvia,
are followed with patients with HIV/AIDS as they should be with every
patient, there is almost no chance of infection, of which physicians are
certainly aware. The ethics of the nontreatment stance are totally unacceptable, particularly in view of the power, profession, and role of healer.

Gender in Medicine: Textbook Examples

Because attitudes and ideas regarding gender expectations are perpetuated through the process of socialization, healers within a society are subject to them like everyone else. Our biases are clearly shown in the language
we use to talk about biology. As Emily Martin (1990) found, immune cells
are described in various biomedical publications as making up an "infan-
try" of "mobile regiments," "snipers," "soldiers," "bodyguards," and even
"killer cells" that "shoot lethal proteins" at enemy invaders (412). In part
due to the historically male make-up of our armed forces, the imagery
evoked is purely masculine. This becomes more apparent when the hierarchy of immune system cells is examined.

As Martin explains, the so-called lower cells—the ones that engulf dying
enemies and clear up debris—are generally described in feminine terms.
The process of forming a pouch for engulfing or eating debris is called
"invagination," and certain biomedical texts actually refer to the pouch as
"vaginal" (1990: 416). Heroic male killer cells shoot enemies, and female
drudges clean up the mess. While there might be many other ways of imaging or talking about what takes place (e.g., as a food chain), and there
is no scientific reason to attribute gender or sex to cells which have neither,
gender imagery is predominant in this discourse, and gender stereotypes
are reinforced each time that we use this discourse in teaching or talking
about the immune system.

Gender stereotypes permeate all levels of the health care system, and can
be found in the interactions between doctors and patients, as well as in
textbooks and laboratories. For example, because masculinity is construed
as nonemotional, many men do not show emotions when they feel them.
Others may not even feel them at all; sometimes, suppressed emotion may
end up being expressed in sickness.

Because women are ranked lower than men in the gender hierarchy, gen-
dered health treatment generally has a more severe and negative impact on
them. For example, physician Robert Wilson (1966) advocated massive
doses of estrogen for women at menopause in order to keep them "feminine" (by which he meant beautiful and young). For Dr. Wilson, the female
sex was defined by their ability to menstruate and their culturally defined
physical beauty, the loss of which rendered them "neuters." Menopause
was considered, by Wilson, a "disease condition" expected to produce dan-

gerous physical and psychological symptoms even though the number of menopausal women actually suffering any bothersome symptoms at all is estimated to be only around 20 to 30 percent (Corea 1977: 266).

Wilson was not an exception. Sociologists Diana Scully and Pauline Bart (1979) reviewed twenty-seven modern gynecological textbooks and found the prevailing stereotypes of women were often expressed in recommendations for diagnosis and treatment. Women were seen as fulfilled only by reproducing, mothering, and looking after their husbands. They were expected to be passive and subservient, and health for women was defined as marriage and childbearing, while deviance from this norm was defined as disease-producing. This has changed in the United States.

The idea that women's bodies (or minds) are defective has been reflected in the fact that women received more prescriptions for medications than men, even for similar problems and conditions (see Corea 1977: 91–95). The disparities in terms of surgical intervention are also notable regarding women. The rate of hysterectomies in America is oddly high, especially when compared to other industrialized countries (Eagan 1994: 23; Payer 1988: 125). It thus appears clear that culture has played and plays a strong part in biomedical decisions. As the culture changes, however, and women become more assertive, differences in treatment of males and females should become more equitable, and there are some indications that this is, indeed, the case (see Abraham 1997).

As with gynecological health, mental health has been defined according to adjustment to culturally constructed roles and expectations. Broverman et al. (1970) questioned a group of psychologists, psychiatrists, and social workers regarding their clinical judgments as to traits that characterize healthy, mature males, females, and (sex unspecified) adults.

There was little difference in expectations for a mature, healthy, competent adult and male. For a mentally healthy female, however, traits given were those that are considered (in our culture) negative and even childlike: submissive, easily influenced, not adventurous, dependent, feelings easily hurt, excitable in a crisis, conceited, subjective, and disliking math and science (Broverman et al. 1970). The mature man was a mature adult; a woman was expected to behave immaturely in order to be considered healthy and mature. As Boverman and colleagues state:

Acceptance of an adjustment notion of health, then, places women in the conflictual position of having to decide whether to exhibit those positive characteristics considered desirable for men and adults, and thus have their "femininity" questioned [or be labeled as maladjusted or even mentally unhealthy or ill] or to behave in the prescribed feminine manner, accept second-class adult status, and possibly live a lie to boot. (1970: 6)

An "adjustment" notion of either physical or mental health must, by definition, be related to the social structure and culture. Adjustment may mean conforming to a socially constructed ideal that supports a particular power structure in the society. Broverman et al. suggest, for example, that black persons who conformed or were "well-adjusted" to the stereotype of the pre–civil rights Negro as passive, docile, child-like, and happy, would be considered healthy, mature adults (1970: 6).

Diagnostic criteria thus reflect attitudes, beliefs, and values instilled in health professionals as they grow up. Enculturation leads to different labeling, diagnoses, and treatment of men and women. Since health care providers are expected to be the experts, their behaviors and actions, and ultimately social and medical policy, in turn support and perpetuate gender and other stereotypes. It is therefore necessary for the providers of health care to examine and correct their own stereotypes and biases.

Gender, Morbidity, and Mortality

Male-female differences are not confined to differences in diagnostic standards. Statistics show real differences in male and female health problems. Women, for example, have higher rates of acute illness such as infectious, respiratory, and digestive problems not related to pregnancy. They also have higher rates of certain chronic, long-term conditions such as hypertension, anemia, colitis, migraine headaches, arthritis, and gallbladder problems. Men have higher rates of accidents and injuries, gout, emphysema, and coronary heart disease. Men also have higher rates of cancer in the youngest and oldest age categories, while women have higher rates between 20 and 55. The chronic problems of men are more likely to lead to death (NCHS 1991).

There are also male-female differences in patterns of health care utilization. Women use health services more often than men, even when maternity services are excluded. Although reasons for this pattern of care-seeking are far from clear, some possibilities include the fact that women employed in lower-paying jobs therefore lose less for time off, plus the fact that they are more aware of health status (especially when they have children), and receive more positive reinforcement for care-seeking. Further, women may feel that it is their duty to care for the sick and so may be more willing than men to bring children in for treatment (Verbrugge 1990).

Men may be more stoic than women about pain or health problems. Women may place a higher value on health, and they may be more willing than males to admit to and acknowledge symptoms and attend to them as well as report them, which is consistent with role expectations (Weiss and Lonnquist 1994: 55–56).

Although women report more illnesses than men, on average, in the United States, they can expect to live almost seven years longer. This holds true across ethnic and socioeconomic groups. Part of the explanation for these differences clearly lies in expectations for gender behavior. Men are more vulnerable to death through violence and accidents than women are (Waldron 1994: 45, 49). To be masculine in America, one takes risks: men's heavier drinking, greater gun use, less safe driving patterns, and higher rates of smoking have significance for male mortality patterns (49). Cross-culturally, more men than women smoke, and in the United States, from one-quarter to three-fifths of the sex difference in mortality due to ischemic heart disease may be related to cigarette smoking (46).

Other attempts to explain the differences in morbidity and mortality include biological or sex-linked differences, such as women's childbearing risks and men's risk for heart disease. Some women do get heart disease, but as Waldron reports, women's lower rate of death from the condition seems to be related to "protective effects of female sex hormones and harmful effects of men's tendency to accumulate fat in the abdominal region" (51). Still, differing trends over time and their historical explanations confirm the heavy influence of social and behavioral factors.

Women's experiences with Caesarean sections neatly demonstrate the influence nonmedical factors have on treatment decisions. The Caesarean operation was named for Julius Caesar, who was said to have been cut from his mother's womb. The operation itself has saved many lives and has helped to reduce both maternal and infant mortality rates. But the increasingly inappropriate use of the operation for nonmedical reasons has become problematic (Annas 1994: 30).

In 1970, the rate of Caesareans in the United States was around 5 percent. The figure leaped to 25 percent by 1988 (Eagan 1994). The advantages of the Caesarean for the physician, as well as the hospital, included more predictable and convenient scheduling of births as well as a larger fee.

Paradoxically, not only have women been inappropriately overmedicated and overtreated, they have also been undermedicated and undertreated. Women have also been seen to "overreact" and to imagine various symptoms. One 1979 university study quoted in Eagan (1994) found that men's reported symptoms (including chest pain, fatigue, headaches, and dizziness) were taken more seriously, generating thorough workups in every case. These symptoms were often dismissed when reported by women (23) (see Abraham 1997 for indications of change).

Irving Zola (1983), when reviewing some previous research on problems of ethnicity in doctor-patient communications, realized that when the males in the population had reported symptoms for which there was no organic cause identified, they were given "nonjudgmental diagnoses," while for females the same types of complaints were noted as either "psychological or of no clinical significance, depending on ethnic group." Zola also observed that all the examining physicians were white males (134).

The Women's Health Movement

It was the women's health movement that provided the impetus to break the vicious cycle of female stereotypes being taught to and then reinforced by the biomedical profession. Growing out of the ferment of the 1960s, the women's health movement was based on a consciousness raised in part by women's health issues of the times. Public debate over the safety of the birth control pill and the related amount of information that should be given to women; the revelations about the dangers of diethylstilbestrol (DES), a drug given to prevent miscarriage that caused vaginal cancer in the daughters of women who had received it; the use of the Dalkon Shield or "copper coil" birth control device, which caused severe infections and sometimes sterility in many users; the revelations of the dangers of uterine cancer from use of estrogen in menopausal women—all mobilized women to ask more questions, demand answers, and educate themselves about their own bodies and health care.

The militancy and activism of the 1970s changed not only women's attitudes, but those of the biomedical profession as well. Women formed health "collectives" that provided education and sometimes care as well. The groundbreaking *Our Bodies, Ourselves* was first published in 1972 by the Boston Women's Health Book Collective and is still in print. The topics cover all areas of women's health from anatomy to sexuality to abortion. The idea was to teach women about themselves as females and not to simply accept biomedicine's (society's) definitions. As Zola (1983) observed, "The women's movement has . . . recently pointed out that the sick role and the labeling of many of their physical issues as sickness has to a very large extent been a way of keeping them in their place" (238).

The relationship of women and their doctors was "deconstructed" (Eagan 1994) as women began to demand information and to refuse having their concerns taken lightly or dismissed. "Some doctors resisted the change; others tried to find a more positive response" (1994: 23). Patients, male as well as female, began to demand a greater participation in decision-making about their health and their health care.

Health Care Workers: The Gender Factor

Possibly the greatest change in male-female relationships has come because of the increasing number of women becoming doctors themselves. In 1970, female physicians constituted 7.6 percent of the total number of doctors in the United States. By 1992, the percentage had risen to 18.1 percent (American Medical Association 1993). This figure will continue to rise as the number of women entering medical school also rises. In 1995, the number of women applying to medical school rose to an unprecedented

42.5 percent of all medical school applicants (*Monthly Forum on Women in Higher Education* 1995: 6–7).

Although in the United States 73 percent of all practicing physicians are still male and 93 percent of nurses are women, things do appear to be changing (*Monthly Forum on Women in Higher Education* 1995: 7). Many women, particularly nurses, are moving into more powerful administrative positions (Fagin 1994: 171). Just how the increasing participation of women will affect the system remains to be seen. The speculation that more women going into biomedicine would result in a more sensitive and caring profession, with improved doctor-patient communication, has not been substantiated. Women physicians have been shown to adopt many of the same values and behaviors as their male counterparts in many situations (Friedman 1994: 8). This testifies to the fact that male and female attributes can be and are learned as appropriate under various conditions, and that medical schools can and must teach students of all genders to truly care for their patients, for themselves, and for each other.

MICRO, MACRO, AND GLOBAL SYSTEMS

Both medical care providers and patients may be greatly affected by the systems and institutions within which they work and receive care. **Macro-level** or institutional, social-structural arrangements determine how, where, what, to whom, and by whom care is delivered (e.g., on the basis of ethnicity, class, or gender); that is, they affect health-related experiences at the **micro** or personal, immediate, and interactive level, which involves the web of interpersonal relationships.

Global systems entail structural arrangements that incorporate not just one society but others as well. Biomedicine, as practiced in various countries, comprises a global system of care. As the world grows smaller and nations and peoples become more interdependent, more and more links connect the micro- and macrolevels with global systems and issues. Macrolevel and global arrangements can have great impacts on health at the personal micro and community levels—impacts often far greater than those that culture per se may have. The connections between and among all three levels of organization may be noted in the following case.

HECTOR VELEZ

Hector Velez, a Mexican immigrant to America diagnosed with cancer, seemingly "made a habit of not showing up for scheduled doctor's appointments and then arriving unexpectedly" (Galanti 1991: 29). Some might argue that Mr. Velez was, in keeping with his culture, acting on a "present time orientation, which is inconsistent with clock time. . . . Someone with a strong present time orientation would tend to get involved in the activity of the moment and not think about the time necessary to get somewhere at a particular hour" (30). Others might explain Mr. Velez's behavior as conditioned by the institutional arrangements for health care in his native country: many clinics in Central America (as well as other parts of the world) do not offer appointments to patients, but allow people to call in at their convenience and wait to be seen.

However, both explanations ignore the larger social structural factors conspiring against Mr. Velez and other people in the lowest economic classes. As Geri-Ann Galanti, who recorded the Velez case, points out, "Many poor people have difficulty getting time off from work to make an appointment. Public transportation is not always reliable. For the poor, life is often a matter of moment-to-moment survival. Advance planning is a luxury that can often be enjoyed only by those with money." And money Mr. Velez did not have. Nor did he have a car, or a phone, or even indoor plumbing. As a social worker investigating his case found out,

> *His home was a broken-down toolshed behind some shacks, which he rented for $75 a month. His shower was a garden hose and his bathroom a neighborhood gas station. He slept on a soiled mattress on the floor and kept his clothes in orange crates that doubled as tables and chairs. He had spent the last three years working as a farm laborer and had recently begun collecting recyclable cans and newspapers to support himself. (Galanti 1991: 30)*

Clearly, more than a present time orientation was behind Mr. Velez' appointment-related behavior; his poverty was key, although his personal behavior was what was reproached. The policies and priorities of macro structures, such as government, which lead to or do not address problems of poverty, provision of education, adequate food supplies, and employment, also underlie his behavior.

Further, Mr. Velez' predicament was related to the global level of international politics and economic conditions in Mexico. International borrowing, debt loads, discriminatory policies, corruption, rising and falling international markets, international political and economic priorities, and interests at home and abroad all may have affected Mr. Velez' needs.

At the global level, the reality of potential catastrophe precipitated by human processes, such as travel, modernization, war, and trade, becomes all too clear when we consider the spread of such diseases as AIDS and Ebola. As the world grows smaller, we cannot escape the possibilities of a global medical disaster, precipitated by social and cultural means as populations come into contact with each other and disturb the ecology. The need, then, is for a cooperative approach that considers the social structural factors that contribute to the dangers and integrates the efforts of various systems to prevent disease and provide care and treatment.

Such an approach must also take into account the structural impact on diverse health needs that arise at different stages of life, such as in protecting children and caring for aging populations. The next chapter examines health from a life course perspective with the aim of generating an appreciation of yet another dimension of human diversity—and similarity.

FOR DISCUSSION

1. What are some of the ways in which social structure determines and influences various health problems in a population?

2. How do the various elements of the social structure help determine who gets sick, who gets care, and what kind of care they get? What significance does "blaming the victim" have in determining causal factors of disease? Which victims are more likely to be blamed? How is blame mitigated by social structure?

3. How are cultural notions used in support of structural barriers or facilitators to health care? How are cultural ideas used to mystify the barriers to care, or even hide their existence in relation to family? Race/ethnic group? Social class? Gender?

4. How can health care clinicians incorporate broader knowledge of families, ethnicity, social class, and gender into more effective care-giving?

3

Health and Illness over the Life Course

Examination of the human life cycle is a good way to look at the interaction of culture and biology. Life cycle stages are often determined by biological events, but each is played out in a cultural context that defines and characterizes it.

[Ferraro, Trevathan, and Levy 1994: 160]

Goal: To identify the uses of the concept of life course and to explore the different perspectives of health and illness in the context of life stages.

Goal: To achieve an awareness of the ways in which the stages of the life course are—and are not—culturally diverse, and how they relate to our health needs and perceptions.

A number of health-related experiences await us on the journey from birth to death. Many are particular to the life stages through which we must pass along the way. Our genetic inheritance provides us each with the basis for certain individual characteristics, talents, and time bombs. Culture, however, will be a major factor in determining whether or not we meet our health potential throughout the life course.

CHARACTERIZING THE LIFE COURSE

The life course provides an excellent framework to discuss and assess questions about differences in needs related to health, illness, and care (Pickin and St. Leger 1993). For example, how are possibilities for health, illness, and responses to illness related to various cultural perceptions of being an adolescent or an adult, or to a society's attitudes and values regarding old age? How do cultural variations in the approach to birth and death relate to giving birth, being born, and dying? And how can an awareness of the cultural context of life stages aid the health care provider as well as the recipient of care?

One of the difficulties in using a concept of life course is deciding where to draw lines dividing one stage from the next. Some studies break the life course down into chronological categories such as "birth to one year," "one to five years," "five to ten years," and so forth. It is more useful here, however, to consider the culturally specific **developmental categories** of infancy, childhood, adolescence, adulthood, and old age.

While individuals in the same stages of the life course have much in common, such as their general biological development and capacities, the various roles they have experienced, and the perspective of the number of years they have lived and have yet to live, life stages are not delimited in exactly the same way cross-culturally. The culturally defined life stage of adulthood, for example, may begin earlier among certain groups (e.g., with first menses or at a certain age, say 13) and later among others (e.g., when a bachelor's degree has been completed or employment first secured). Some of the life stage guidelines deemed important in one culture are deemed inconsequential in another; even the recognition of particular phases as life stages can differ cross-culturally. For example, the time after death when one becomes an ancestor is not a life stage for the biomedical clinician, but it is for some Buddhists (LaFleur 1992).

Further, to conceive of events happening in stages implies delimited events rather than a life continuum, and that each designated stage has a norm. Anything outside the norm may be viewed as abnormal and thus subject to negative labeling and medical or social intervention. Relating to biomedical practice, Stein (quoted in Dossey 1991: 122) observed that "the physician may hide behind the metaphor of the 'stage' instead of confronting the unique person to whom these [stage labels] apply." And as Atchley (1994) notes, "The life course in reality is composed of a great many alternative routes to alternative destinations" (155); this makes normative sequences essentially unrealistic.

Still, various periods in the life course have specific ramifications in terms of our risks and possibilities of illness. In addition, our needs and vulnerabilities at any stage and how they are addressed can be and are mitigated, reduced, enhanced, and changed by cultural and structural factors and variables.

PREGNANCY AND CHILDBIRTH: THE BEGINNING

Culture is relevant to us even before we are born. Various cultural factors can affect the fetus in its development and potential, particularly the health and well-being of the mother. Her poverty, illness, isolation, voluntary and involuntary exposure to toxic substances, stress and disease, accident and violence—all may affect the outcome of pregnancy for the baby, the mother, and the entire family.

The **perinatal** stage covers the period of late pregnancy up to a year after birth, when babies tend to be most vulnerable. More than half of all infant deaths are due to four factors: disorders due to low birth weight, congenital anomalies (birth defects), sudden infant death syndrome (SIDS), and respiratory distress that results from underdeveloped lungs as in prematurity (U.S. Department of Health and Human Services 1992: 9)—again, all may be related to sociocultural factors.

Low birth weight (LBW)—that is, weight at birth of less than 2,500 grams—affects about 7 percent of all live births and is the "greatest single hazard to infant health" (U.S. Department of Health and Human Services 1992: 9). Very low birth weights of less than 1,500 grams may result in such developmental disabilities as cerebral palsy, autism, mental retardation, and vision and hearing impairments; this is especially tragic because LBW is, for the most part, preventable. Culturally related risk factors include lack of prenatal care, maternal smoking, use of alcohol or drugs, and pregnancy before age 18 (10).

Maternal smoking is particularly worrisome as it has been linked to 23 to 30 percent of all LBW births in the United States (Kleinman and Madans 1985). It has been suggested that "If all pregnant women refrained from smoking, fetal and infant deaths would be reduced by approximately 10 percent, saving about 4,000 infants per year" (U.S. Department of Health and Human Services 1992: 11). About 25 percent of pregnant women smoke throughout their pregnancy, with women in the lowest age and socioeconomic groups most likely to do so. Accordingly, LBW is associated with low socioeconomic status and educational level (both associated with poverty); black infants are twice as likely as white infants to be LBW (10).

Birth defects may also be related to various types of social and environmental factors. **Fetal alcohol syndrome (FAS)**, for example, which produces congenital anomalies, stems from excessive alcohol consumption by the mother and a similar syndrome can be found in the babies of drug-addicted mothers. FAS may be manifested in brain damage, facial deformities, and growth and central nervous system dysfunctions. FAS affects from one to three infants per 1,000 live births and may be higher in some populations than others (U.S. Department of Health and Human Services 1992: 10). Other common birth defects, one-fourth of which are due to genetic factors and many of which result in death or long-term disabilities, include malformations of the brain and spine and heart defects. In light of the consequences of FAS, there should be more attention in the medical community to signs of substance abuse in pregnant patients.

Maternal behavior is too often blamed for these and related problems; as stated in chapter 2, the conditions and behavioral implications of poverty must be considered in any discussion of causes and preventive strategies. Women who have little education, cannot afford to adequately feed themselves and their families, cannot afford child care, are uninsured and have little or no access to health care (including prenatal care), and who, if addicted to alcohol or drugs, have no access to substance abuse treatment programs, cannot be expected to remedy the ills of poor birth outcomes by themselves. It is hoped that future research can tell us more about ways to break the cycle (see Singer et al. 1992). We also need much more research on the role of men, the influence of passive and active smoking, domestic violence, and substance abuse by the male on outcome of pregnancy.

Prenatal Care

Since most of these problems are preventable, various forms of intervention may be necessary and desirable to protect babies' and mothers' health and well-being. Therefore, the most important consideration before birth, and one that relates to education and cultural factors, is prenatal care. Education is an essential part of prenatal, as well as postnatal care, and cultural sensitivity and awareness is a necessary part of any prenatal or postnatal care program. Such programs should also involve fathers when this can be done without alienating the target community. It should be recognized that in some cultural groups, especially where levels of sex segregation are high, the father is proscribed from participation in certain activities involving pregnancy and birth.

Proper prenatal care can have a positive effect on birth outcome, particularly for low-income and high-risk women (U.S. Department of Health and Human Services 1992: 12). Even so, since 1980, the proportion of women receiving this care in the first three months of pregnancy for all ethnic groups has not increased (12). This is especially ironic in view of broad attempts to contain health costs. For every case where low birth weight is prevented by prenatal care, the system saves between $14,000 and $30,000 in associated costs (12).

One of the most basic and grave errors made in political, as well as in social and medical, discourse on prenatal care is the culturally influenced failure to consider mother-to-be and fetus as a unit: if mother and fetus are considered separately—which a culture valuing individualism may encourage if the fetus is seen as an individual—it is possible for an adversarial relationship to develop in which the question simply becomes one of whose rights prevail (Johnsen 1987). This is evident in the U.S. abortion debate.

The issue of autonomy has arisen in numerous legal challenges regarding where to draw the line for maternal responsibility and fetal rights. For example, statutes have even allowed children to sue their mothers for behaviors or actions while pregnant that may have adversely affected the child's development prior to birth (Johnsen 1987).

Technological capabilities such as intrauterine surgery have raised questions as to who is really the doctor's patient—the mother or the fetus. Such a question could only arise in a particular cultural context; here, gender power structures and technological ideals are at play (see Davis-Floyd 1992). If the mother refuses such surgery, is she guilty of potential harm to the fetus? Johnsen (1987) notes that women make countless decisions that create some minimal risk of harm, as in driving a car or even in wearing seat belts. Further, we do not force someone not pregnant to undergo a medical procedure for the good of another, even for a child. Fetal rights laws ignore the fact that the woman cannot walk away from the fetus to avoid legal restrictions and liabilities. Pregnancy presents a completely unique situation, both medically and legally.

The issues raised could take us far beyond the focus of this chapter. Nonetheless, the points considered are strongly related to medical decision-making and cultural attitudes and values. It is always much easier to "blame the victim" than to recognize the relationship of social structure, including political values, economic barriers, and social pressures, as the root cause of many health and social problems.

The Culture of Childbirth

Pregnancy and childbirth, so essential to human survival, have always and everywhere been surrounded by an aura of mystery. While this aura will be larger or smaller depending on cultural context, because it is potentially dangerous (as well as life-affirming), birth everywhere is "treated and marked as a life crisis event and as such it entails a multitude of beliefs and rituals meant to help both mother and child and sometimes the entire family or community pass unharmed through this period of danger" (Jordan 1993: 3–4).

While even in very early ethnographies accounts of birth rituals can be found, little was actually known about the female experience of pregnancy and childbirth or women's secret procreative knowledge until recently. This is because anthropology was for so long a bastion of men who could not, in most cultures, be present at birth, let alone participate in women's culture. So it was not until female anthropologists were able to observe and chronicle birthing practices and knowledge from the woman's perspective that much of our present information was gained (Romalis 1981: 9).

In 1978, Brigitte Jordan proposed that birth, a "universal biological function," is embedded in a "culture-specific social matrix" (Jordan 1993: 48). This matrix entails many interactional aspects. The local conceptualization or cultural definition of birth, which will include ideas about who should do it, when, and why, is one feature; birth also features pain and pain management, preparation (including formal or informal education—or the expectation of no instruction at all), attendants and social support systems, a territory or place of action, and technologies or artifacts. Importantly, the latter can determine birth position as well as limit the participation of the birthing mother in her own delivery.

Women cross-culturally give birth in a number of positions, the most effective of which harness the power of gravity to assist in the expulsion of the fetus. Often, someone behind the woman supports her laboring body. Sitting, squatting, kneeling, and standing are popular positions. In a recent study comparing position preferences, the supported squat was most popular by far. These women reported all-around better birth experiences with easier pushing and less pain (Jordan 1993: 85).

Notwithstanding, the American hospital delivery table is constructed in such a way that the only possible way a woman can give birth is lying on her back, in what is called a lithotomy position. The tables have no foot end; women's feet are put up in stirrups. This position decreases the size of the pelvic outlet and puts undue pressure on a woman's pulmonary and cardiac systems, lowering oxygen supply to the fetus. Contractions are weaker and pushing is harder because gravity can be of no aid. Vaginal and perineal tearing are more likely, as is the need for pain medication and labor-inducing chemicals. Further, as there is no space on the delivery table for it, the attending physician is forced to cut the cord to the placenta immediately, which means that the infant does not receive about 25 percent of the blood that it would otherwise take in (Jordan 1993: 84, 86).

In addition to position, the distribution of decision-making rights and the ownership of authoritative medical knowledge are key. For example, in America, where the birthing mother has, with few exceptions, neither total control over decisions nor authority, a woman desiring pain medication may have to "produce the appropriate display of pain experience" to convince the attendant of her need for relief. This "adds to the comparatively high level of noise and hysteria in American obstetric wards but must also provide powerful feedback to increase the subjective experience of pain" (Jordan 1993: 53). In Sweden, by contrast, where pain medication is available on request, "the atmosphere is one of quiet, intense concentration rather than vocal panic and despair" (53).

A huge diversity in birth customs and beliefs exists, although some universal themes and obvious symbols surround the event (Romalis 1981). These include the themes of human continuity and women's power to give life (or nature's power to do so). Some universally potent symbols related to and often referred to in birth ritual cross-culturally are blood, water, milky substances, snakes, rope or cord, and eggs. Blood refers to menses, life blood, and the actual bloodiness of childbirth; water refers to amniotic fluid and drinking water, as well as water for irrigation; milky substances are associated with breast and genital secretions; snakes shed their old skins and have newly regenerated ones underneath, as well as resembling the penis and the umbilical cord, which is itself represented in rope or cord, also representative of family ties; eggs symbolize the continuity of life, re-birth, spring, and life potential. More specific meanings will also be found in each culture, where local beliefs as well as environmental and historical conditions will lead members to particularize the connotations of each symbol.

In Jamaica, where heavy ritual action is generally not undertaken unless there are problems with a pregnancy, simple preventive steps in which simple symbolism is manipulated are the norm (Sobo 1993). For instance, a mother-to-be avoids stepping over ropes or vines to keep the fetus from becoming entwined in its umbilical cord. She does not tip her head back too far when drinking to avoid suffocating the fetus. A mother's food cravings must be met or her child's body will be marked; however, too much of one food can affect fetal development. Similar practices have been recorded for many cultural groups.

Superficially superstitious practices may be based in common sense understandings about fetal development and about the effect that actions in one realm may have on another. As long as such practices do no harm, they can support a client's sense of well-being, and they should not be discouraged by health practitioners. In fact, by making a mother feel good about taking culturally recommended proactive measures, other prenatal care practices, such as those promoted by biomedicine, can be encouraged. The same holds true for postnatal practice. Supporting an African Caribbean woman who wants to pin a piece of red cloth or ribbon on her newborn's vest to ward off evil can help build trust and encourage her in taking up biomedically effective health-promotion practices.

Some birth rituals may include the provision of social and emotional support during labor and birth. Among the Maya in Yucatan, who give birth in their homes, along with the midwife and the woman's mother, the father-to-be is present to support his partner both physically (he sits behind her) and emotionally. It is important for him to witness her pain (Jordan 1993). In American hospitals, strangers are often the only witnesses.

In some cultures, the man participates in pregnancy itself, experiencing morning sickness and other symptoms. Pregnancy is, then, not a private individual condition, but one that affects the parents together. The anthropological term for this is *couvade*. Couvade signifies and tightens conjugal bonds and gives a man what Moore et al. call "cultural confirmation" (1987 [1980]: 118) of paternity. Reproductive rituals ensure the well-being of all. They also help cement social ties and reinforce social structural family arrangements.

The Biomedical View

Biomedicine views pregnancy and especially childbirth as medical events. Through **medicalization** of childbirth, physicians tend to define and treat the condition of pregnancy as abnormal—a condition that only they can manage.

While millions of babies are born successfully without intervention of physicians, biomedicine has enjoyed great success in reducing the maternal mortality rate (Friedman 1994: 3). Women died from complications of childbirth at high rates before surgical procedures, such as the use of the forceps, to remove fetal obstructions were invented. Before the germ theory became widely accepted, however, physician-attended births frequently ended with the mother's death from childbed fever, or puerperal sepsis, because doctors did not recognize the need for cleanliness.

Childbed fever had not been a widely experienced problem prior to the advent of hospitalization during birth. It was Austrian physician Ignaz Semmelweis who first noticed, in the 1840s, a link between unwashed hands and the disease. He saw that, in his hospital, women attended by doctors had a rate of childbed fever five times that of those attended by midwives. Semmelweis ordered hand washing with disinfectant, and a dramatic decrease in the disease was seen (Jordan 1993: 51).

While hand washing was clearly necessary, Davis-Floyd writes that "the removal of birth to the hospital has resulted in a proliferation of rituals surrounding this natural physiological event more elaborate than any heretofore known in the 'primitive' world. These rituals, also known as 'standard procedures for normal birth' work to effectively convey the core values of American society" (1992: 1–2).

Such rituals include shaving the pubic area, giving the birthing woman an enema, and prohibiting any food intake. While these procedures are rationalized as promoting sanitation in the controlled birth arena, they actually can lead to higher rates of infection, for instance through nicks made during shaving. A lack of nourishment saps energy and subsequently lengthens labor, as well as increasing the acidity of any vomit. Enemas, which can be very painful, decrease neither the likelihood of elimination during labor nor the incidence of fecal contamination (Davis-Floyd 1992: 83, 85, 89).

Other ritual procedures, such as attaching women to umbilicus-like intravenous drips and fetal monitors, limit their mobility and confine them to the lithotomy position, which can prolong labor and necessitate further medical intervention in a domino effect (Davis-Floyd 1992: 94–95, 106). IV glucose drips can even lower women's tolerance to pain, necessitating more medication (93).

Another way to understand American birth ritual is through an examination of the experiences of nurse midwives (Rothman 1994: 104–12). Nurses' training is well grounded in the biomedical model. When becoming midwives, however, nurses are exposed to anomalies that challenge biomedical knowledge of childbirth. The differences primarily involve biomedically defined stages of the birth process, each of which has a statistically, biomedically estimated norm of time allotted.

Hospital births are speeded up when a particular stage is seen as taking too long. Intervention may be justified biomedically, for example as minimizing danger and discomfort to mother and baby. However, the number of hospital deliveries to be processed in a given period of time is a prime factor in the decision to intervene. If a woman's body's birth timetable is too short or too long, the routine of the hospital is upset; deviations are unthinkable (Rothman 1994: 111).

Thus, when nurse midwives witness healthy out-of-hospital births in women who do not conform to the biomedical timetable, they begin to challenge the biomedical model itself. The range of "normal" becomes much broader and individualized (Rothman 1994).

INFANCY

Infant Death

In spite of biomedicine's benefits, the infant mortality rate in the United States is higher than in Japan, Sweden, Canada, Germany, and several other industrialized countries (Adams and Benson 1991). However, also within the United States, infant mortality is higher for some groups than others; these rates are another indicator of social inequality. Infant mortality rates have historically been about twice as high for black babies as for white babies in the United States, and the gap has remained (Rice 1990: 74). Since Blacks are overrepresented in the poor population, and the poor have the highest infant mortality rates across all groups, the major factor here is not race or ethnicity, but poverty (Polednak 1989). So, infant mortality rates reflect a broader social reality.

A problem possibly related to family structure and modern lifestyle, **Sudden Infant Death Syndrome (SIDS)**, accounts for about one-third of U.S. infant deaths after the first month of life (U.S. Department of Health and Human Services 1992: 10). Causes are not known, but SIDS is thought to be tied to genetics, maternal smoking and drug use, young age of mother, parent-infant sleeping arrangements, and infections late in pregnancy (10). Recent research suggests that sleep position, with the baby lying on its stomach, may account for some cases of SIDS (Taylor et al. 1996).

Immunization

Up until the early twentieth century, infectious disease was the major cause of death for children in all societies (Cockburn 1963). The turnabout was related to the invention of a range of immunization techniques and products by which vaccinated children were protected from what were heretofore killer diseases, such as polio and whooping cough. Uninnocu-lated children—and the ethnic or class groups they mainly represented—were culturally transformed into public health threats.

Despite their potential benefits, present-day immunization efforts some-times fall flat in the face of understandings about some of the ingredients used to manufacture immunization compounds (e.g., blood serum from cattle or horses). Members of certain groups, therefore, in keeping with their cultural beliefs about what should and should not enter the body, refuse to be immunized. Some also shun immunization because of beliefs about penetration of body boundaries (e.g., the skin).

Sometimes, merely the provision of alternate routes of innoculation (e.g., oral ingestion) or of preparations without any offending ingredients, or patiently explaining that what the client thinks is in the vaccine actually is not, is enough to change a "no" to a "yes."

Nutritional Concerns

In addition to exposure to infectious diseases often spread through cul-tural practices, babies are vulnerable to other culture-linked hazards. For example, infants are vulnerable to infections and malnutrition that can be prevented by breast milk, which provides antibodies and proper nourish-ment. When mothers no longer nurse their young, due to the development and use of infant formulas, infants can lose some degree of this naturally conferred immunity.

Another reason to breastfeed, especially in poor populations, is that as long as breasts and especially nipples are wiped clean before nursing, di-arrheal diseases can be better avoided if no formula is given. Formula often is mixed with unclean water and given in unsterilized bottles or cups. Con-taminated water and utensils can trouble the gut, and malnutrition results when food is not kept in the digestive tract long enough to be absorbed. Further, formula often is diluted by poor mothers who need to stretch it, meaning that nutrients taken in would not, even if absorbed, be enough to provide a good nutritive start for the infant (Moore et al. 1987 [1980]: 124).

While this can be a problem in industrialized societies, in developing countries, where infant mortality is much higher with limited or no access to care, the marketing and distribution of infant formula can have disas-terous effects. For infants who do not breastfeed in these countries, the death rate is ten to fifteen times greater in the first three to four months than for breastfeeding babies (Sokol 1992: 9). Impoverished infants in ghet-tos, barrios, and poverty-stricken rural areas in America are as much at risk and vulnerable to many of the same hazards as children in economi-cally underdeveloped nations.

The Trials of Childhood

Childhood is generally a time of learning and anticipatory socialization for the life ahead. It is also the stage at which good health habits can be developed, such as adequate practices of diet, exercise, dental care, and body awareness. Now that major infectious diseases are generally under control, the major cause of death among children is injuries—primarily unintentional injuries occurring from motor vehicle crashes (U.S. Department of Health and Human Services 1992: 12). Preventive care needs to go beyond immunizations and recognition and treatment of early problems to include raising awareness of possible accidents, such as poisoning and drowning, and encouraging proper use of automobile seat belts or restraining devices.

Childhood illness and accidents are strongly associated with poverty and low educational levels. These can make proper nutrition, exercise, and preventive health care impossible. Since resulting health problems may produce long-term conditions such as mental retardation, learning disorders, behavioral problems, and sensory impairments, "an accurate profile of the health of U.S. children . . . must also consider emotional, psychological, and learning problems, the social and environmental risks to which they are related, and the total costs to the Nation" (U.S. Department of Health and Human Services 1992: 12).

A tremendous problem for children across cultures is intentional injury and abuse. Abuse includes neglect, withholding or delaying medical treatment, and outright violent attack. While violence affects us at all levels of the life course, abuse of children is particularly deplorable because of the power disparity in the adult-child relationship. The effects of child abuse last a lifetime and impact on victims' abilities to function as healthy adults (see Widom 1989).

More than 1 million U.S. children are abused each year, and in many cases the abuse is never reported (Westat, Inc. 1988). Physical abuse is most common, with emotional and sexual abuse following. Much abuse is found in poor families; however, "any correlation between abuse and poverty is biased by the fact that the behavior of the poor is more likely to be reported in official records than that of members of other classes, who are better equipped to conceal their activities" (Kornblum and Julian 1995: 211).

Although domestic abuse seems to be most common in industrialized nations, it also exists in other societies, including small-scale ones (Korbin 1987; Soroka and Bryjak 1995: 315–17). Developing nations, due to greater concerns over disease and malnutrition, are only beginning to see mistreatment of children as an issue to be addressed (Korbin 1987).

Treatment of children should always be understood within a cultural context, as should the definition of "harm." However, argues Korbin (1987), "Any practice, whether collective or individual, that compromises children's development and survival must be critically considered. Practices that inflict potential physical or psychic pain and harm on all children, or all children in particular categories, must be subjected to empirical tests of harm and not judged on an implicit or explicit ethnocentric basis" (29). Harming children (like harming anyone) must not be accepted as a culturally relative practice justified by tradition.

Korbin states that "cultural competence challenges ethnocentric beliefs about what is good for children or what is abusive and neglectful. It also furthers knowledge of the circumstances under which child abuse and neglect are most likely to occur and, in turn, most likely to be prevented" (1987: 35).

Several factors placing children at risk for abuse are identified across cultures: deformities or handicaps and multiple or difficult births, which may be interpreted as malevolent or inauspicious; culturally defined illigitimacy; gender preferences; rapid socioeconomic and sociocultural change; urbanization; stress; unemployment; and poverty. The fact that immigrant children may become knowledgeable and acculturate to a new environment more rapidly than parents and become less obedient and compliant also may come into play (Korbin 1987).

The AMA provides medical guidelines to physicians for identifying and handling domestic abuse. Health care providers must comply with laws where abuse is suspected, but they can also inform themselves regarding supportive networks and agencies such as churches, shelters, and other advocates for battered women and children, and provide appropriate referrals. Additional resources and referrals may be necessary since children are themselves becoming more involved as protagonists in violent behavior, creating further problems for providing care.

Since the traditional biomedical system addresses cure rather than prevention, the focus is on treating conditions after they occur. The preventability of many childhood medical problems vividly illustrates the inadequacy of this type of approach. Physicians, however, are beginning to participate as advocates of preventive programs. The AMA and other medical organizations have thrown their weight behind a number of public health campaigns and related legislation. Their goals have included the prevention of cigarette smoking in children, the eliminations of dangerous exposure to second-hand smoke, and the promotion of seat belt use in automobiles.

ADOLESCENCE

Violence is not confined to children; adolescents also are abused, and they abuse others. In our society, this is tied in part to the cultural view of adolescence as a time for risk-taking and dramatics. However, as Margaret Mead (1963 [1928]) showed so many years ago, adolescence need not be a time of great "sturm und drang"—it certainly was not stormy for the Samoan adolescents involved in her research. For them, "adolescence represented no period of crisis or stress" (95), partly because of the "general casualness" (117) of Samoan culture and partly because of a cultural value on conflict avoidance.

Despite cultural differences, adolescence "is everywhere associated with pubertal events such as menstruation, the appearance of secondary sexual features . . . or general changes in body conformation," write Schlegel and Barry (1991: 198–99), whose major cross-cultural study of adolescence was the first of its kind. After systematically investigating compiled data from 186 societies, the researchers concluded that adolescence is indeed a universal life stage, albeit one that varies according to a group's economic, familial, and social structural organization.

Adolescence also varies by gender: generally it lasts longer for boys than for girls, who may enter the status of adult earlier than boys do, through pregnancy or marriage (Schlegel and Barry 1991: 12). Girls also experience their growth spurt (e.g., in height) and reproductive maturation closer together in time than do boys (Moore et al. 1987 [1980]: 138). And they have the very demarcated experience of menarche, the first menstrual flow, while for boys physical puberty is a more nebulous event. In Europe and the United States, menarche now occurs about two years earlier than it did 100 years ago. Worldwide, it occurs earlier in urban areas and among the wealthy. These trends seem to be linked to better nutrition and increased body fat (139–40). Emotional maturity, however, may be less developed.

Youthful Risk Taking

Adolescence is a time of exploration, and this sometimes involves risk taking. This can be noted with initiation of sexual activity. By the age of 16, 17 percent of American girls and 29 percent of American boys have had sexual intercourse (Hechinger 1992: 3). In 1990, 66 percent of Massachusetts youths were sexually active, an 11 percent increase over 1986 figures (Hingson and Strunin 1992: 20). Only 37 percent of the sexually active youths in this study reported consistent condom use (20). (Reported behavior is not necessarily reflected in actual practice.)

Without barrier protection, youths are vulnerable to a range of sexually transmitted conditions, including pregnancy and HIV infection. Factual education alone is obviously not the answer. There seems to be little relation between knowledge of sexual risks and decreased risky behavior (Hingson and Strunin 1992: 24). This is in part because adolescents in America are socialized to take sexual risks. There are many cultural reasons for doing so, one being that such behavior confers status and self-esteem (see Sobo 1995). It may also not be perceived as "risky."

Further, what is risky in one situation might not be as risky in another.

For example, while pregnant teens in middle-class neighborhoods might have little practical experience in childcare and might have many opportunities for further education, an inner-city teen will have spent a great deal of time caring for others' babies and will probably not even have the same educational chances as middle-class girls who bear children will consequently lose.

Youthful risk-taking in the United States goes beyond sex to include substance abuse—the use of drugs, tobacco, or alcohol. About one in five high-school seniors uses illicit drugs (this figure excludes school dropouts, among whom drug use may be higher) (U.S. Department of Health and Human Resources 1992: 18), and about one in five high-school seniors report that they smoke (17). Driving is also, for many youths, a symbol of their increasing maturity and so is an eagerly approached activity. It also is one that frequently entails risk-taking. Automobile accidents are a major cause of death and disability among adolescents (U.S. Department of Health and Human Resources 1992: 17).

While tobacco is a problem, alcohol use is particularly high among American adolescents and may be connected to the automobile accidents. About 60 percent of high-school seniors reported drinking in the previous month in a 1989 survey; 33 percent reported drinking heavily—having five or more drinks on one occasion—in the previous two weeks. Heavy drinking also was reported by 28 percent of eighth graders and 38 percent of tenth graders in a 1987 survey (U.S. Department of Health and Human Resources 1992: 17).

Intervention must take place in the early grades, and it should go beyond simple factual health messages to address broader cultural issues that surround risky activities. For example, teens could be reminded that smoking causes bad breath, which others find offensive. The opinions of others, however, could also promote the habit: some teens smoke to stay thin. Because of cultural values, the fear of fat may override any fears about personal offense or even possible lung cancer (Hechinger 1992: 11). Education for a healthy diet, as well as to build self-esteem, may do the most good here.

Care after the fact involves recognition, sensitivity, building trust, and referral skills in the health care provider. Confidentiality also must be assured; adolescents' fear of breaches in confidentiality may keep them from telling practitioners about their substance use or about other sensitive matters. In a Massachusetts study, 25 percent of high-school students reported that they would forego health care in some situations if they thought that their parents might find out (Cheng et al. 1993: 1404).

Suicide and Sexual Identity

Another major cause of death among youths is suicide, which generally has complex social roots. Suicide is the little-known but leading cause of death for gay male, lesbian, bisexual, and transsexual youth (Messina 1992: 1). Suicide often stems from a crisis related to the adolescent's self-identification as being nonheterosexual; U.S. cultural attitudes make such identification problematic. Because of this, gay and lesbian youth are two to three times more likely to attempt suicide than heterosexual youth, and such suicide attempts are "more serious and more lethal than those of their heterosexual peers" (Messina 1992: 1). Health care providers may have an impact on this problem through showing sensitivity and concern, rather than denial or condemnation for nonheterosexual identities in their young patients.

ADULTHOOD

Responsibility for Self and Others

Adults have more opportunity than infants, children, adolescents, or old people to take responsibility for their health. Many of the leading causes of death in adults are preventable, often through lifestyle changes. The decline in rates of coronary heart disease and stroke deaths, both of which have dropped by about half since 1970, is in a large part due to a decrease in cigarette smoking and an increased attention to diet and to controlling high blood pressure. Over the same time period, adult automobile accident death rates declined by about one-third. This was due to more seatbelt use, less alcohol use, and lowered speed limits. Social and behavioral changes—and cultural changes that supported them—thus affected adults' health status (U.S. Department of Health and Human Services 1992: 19). Also during adulthood, poor or toxic working conditions, high stress levels, alcohol and tobacco use, depression, and despair all may take their toll, especially on poor and homeless adults.

Still, adults have more autonomy than youths and more authority, enabling them to control health policies and laws that can affect specific populations or society in general. Adults can, in principle, make or repeal laws dealing with pollution, risky behavior, or safe food supplies and consumer goods. However, they also face various health problems particular to their life stage, as well as those related to earlier behaviors and lifestyles.

Menopause: Biology and Culture

Gender differences in the meaning of adulthood are perhaps more profound than cultural differences in the achievements by which one becomes a social adult. In some societies, women who are social adults still have only the rights of children and can make few decisions for themselves.

In some cultures, this changes after women undergo menopause (e.g., among the Hua; see Meigs 1983: 5, 48, 67), the logic being that now that they do not menstruate and cannot bear children they are more like men and should therefore have similar rights. Of course, in other contexts, post-menopausal women may be seen not so much "as good as" men, but rather as "lesser" women.

Because of cultural norms for female bodies, postmenopausal women in the United States may interpret changes, such as facial hair growth or a lowering of vocal pitch (Katchadourian 1978: 47), as masculinization. Infertility may be distressing for women in certain cultural contexts, where women's value hinges on their childbearing function. But it also can come as a relief, in that the fear of pregnancy is abated; some women experience heightened erotic responsiveness at this time (47).

Menopause itself is a very nebulous process. The label of "menopause," however, constructs what is partly a social transition as a purely biological transition. Biomedical specialists define menopause technically as the occurrence of the last menstrual period, making it an "event in time" (Kaufert 1986: 333). However, women cross-culturally experience it as a process that takes place *over* time, and they use a "self-anchoring definition" (333) of menopause, seeing themselves as menopausal when there has been a change in their bodily patterns—for example, in the menstrual cycle.

The biomedical definition of menopause is used in a scientific context, as a woman's last menstrual period is relatively stable and objective across populations. Signs and symptoms are more ambiguous, however, and because a woman's own definitions may be equally valid, the physician's role should not be to define, but to distinguish between the pathological and the nonpathological in the client (Kaufert 1986: 76).

The physician also needs to bear in mind that there are many reasons besides menopause that might account for menstrual changes. Indeed, as Patricia Kaufert notes, "A model based on the well-nourished women of the white middle class is clearly inappropriate to societies where women are frequently malnourished or constantly overburdened by pregnancy or physical or psychological stress. Under these conditions menstruation becomes sparse and irregular well before the expected age of menopause" (1986: 335).

Although the average age of 50 is remarkably universal for onset of menopause, a survey of thirty societies revealed that only in two societies besides the United States was the event seen as a major physical and emotional loss (Bart 1969). The accompanying symptoms of distress found in the United States are not even noted in many other societies, such as in India (Flint 1975).

Biomedically, not only women but also men undergo "menopause." For men, who do not have such a visible sign of fecundity as the menstrual period, menopause is "a far more dubious entity" (Katchadourian 1978: 47). As with women, hormone balances gradually change. Testicular function gradually declines, and men experience an attendant loss in potency and fertility. In the United States, these changes are not culturally or even often biomedically recognized; they challenge sociocultural concepts of both masculinity and femininity. It is significant that there is no biomedical specialty for male sexual or reproductive problems, which are instead included under the specialty of urology.

Notwithstanding, men, like women, can remain sexually active into old age. Cultural values, however, tend to characterize older men and women past childbearing age as asexual (Stanford 1977). Any interest manifested in sex, even in the face of research by Kinsey, Pomeroy, and Martin (1948; 1953) and later by Masters and Johnson (1966), is still too often seen as abnormal by the biomedical profession, as well as by society.

THE AGING POPULATION

Growing Old Culturally

Aging is unpopular in the United States. Although the number of older citizens now comprises about 14 percent of the population and is increasing rapidly, the cultural emphasis is still on the youthful image. Products are constantly emerging in the market place to erase or minimize wrinkles, color or replace hair, provide boundless energy, improve memory, and boost sexual prowess and performance. Some of these products and procedures, such as plastic surgery, face lifts, varicose vein removal, tummy tucks, and liposuction, are obtained within or from the biomedical institution. The market for such treatments and services is expanding as the aging population continues to grow.

The fact that more and more people are living into their seventies and eighties, plus the unprecedented rise in birth rates after World War II (the baby boom cohort), means that we will see a large bulge in the retirement population somewhere between 2015 and 2030 (Atchley 1994: 44–45). The resulting changes in proportions in age categories will have profound consequences for the restructuring of health care.

Those age 85 and up (the old-old) will be the fastest growing group, reaching 19 million by 2050 (U.S. Bureau of the Census 1993a). There will be more elderly women, because (unless the ratios change) women outlive men by about seven years. The old-old (mostly women) will also be more likely than others to live in nursing homes and to have substantial disabilities and extremely limited financial resources. Even though at present most older people do receive care and assistance from spouses and families, that arrangement may change. More people do not marry or have children, families have grown smaller, and people's human and financial resources have shrunk (see chapter 2).

Although aging is not a disease any more than is childhood, adolescence, or adulthood, the last years of our lives carry a higher risk of chronic ailments, some of which may have taken root at an earlier time in the life course. The most common cause of death in elderly American adults, male and female, is now heart disease, followed by cancer and stroke (Kart 1990: 69). Chronic problems require a different type of medical care; they generally cannot be cured, but must be managed through cooperation of physician and patient, with family, on a long-term basis.

In addition, the quantity of life has been extended more for some groups than others. Aging in ethnic minority groups may have a different significance than it does for the mainstream, but the same social structure that allows discrimination and unequal opportunity for members of minority groups has a direct impact on the possibilities of such people reaching old age, and on the physical, mental, social and economic condition of those who get there.

A lifetime of poverty and distress, including a work history of part-time, low-paying, physically demanding or hazardous jobs, with few benefits and perhaps many periods without work, will lead to more health problems and fewer resources at old age. Thus, being old and poor, or old and poor and female or old and poor and female and minority, compounds all the problems of aging. Treating the aging population will be a major challenge for the health care system.

Cultural Meanings of Age: The Mainstream

Treatment for the elderly requires a knowledge of related cultural factors and attitudes that also influence the types and rates of illness, both physical and mental, as well as causes of death in all cultural groups. In many societies, wisdom and authority are attributed to the elderly who, through life experience, have gained social standing and achieved the right to respect. They may also be seen as a major resource in teaching others how to understand the world and to survive.

Cultural views of aging in the United States are tied to historical and social structural factors as well as to related ideals and values. General negative connotations of aging came with modernization. Before the American Revolution, older, free, white males from the appropriate social class owned property, directed the family, and therefore had much control within the community and held advantages in trade, politics, and religion. There were fewer elderly; age was considered granted by God's favor and therefore venerated.

Modernization theory points to a concomitant loss of roles for the elderly. The wisdom of age becomes obsolete, civil authority is dispersed to younger citizens, and there is an expansion of wealth and trade. Land ownership becomes less important with growth of industry and urbanization (Cowgill 1972).

Atchley (1994), however, proposes that it is social ideology more than objective reality that has influenced our perceptions of aging. The ideals of equality undermined the moral basis for a hierarchical, age-graded society even before that equality was declared in law. Further, as modernization increased its pace, older people were culturally cast as obsolete.

In any case, with modernization, improved standards of living and medical care extended life expectancy. More people began to live longer. By the 1930s, social security was created to provide a motivation for retirement, freeing up jobs for younger citizens as well as offering a cushion for retirees. Ironically, social security contributed to a vision of the elderly as less capable and unable to manage by themselves (Atchley 1994).

In many ways, the biomedical institution also contributed to the developing cultural view of aging as a time of increasing dependency and decrepitude, with expectations of aches and pains, memory loss, and other concomitant conditions. Biological research on the aging process characterized it as natural decline and degeneration (see Atchley 1994).

Paradoxically, modernization also produced better diets, better general living conditions, and longer life expectancy. In response to the needs and demands of a growing elderly population, new discoveries and research on aging have contributed to a healthier, more active, and hence even larger population of citizens at the far end of life. The older population increasingly has refused to accept aging as obsolescence. The old-old, however, are and will be the most fragile and the most ill.

Aging Outside of the Mainstream

From a multicultural perspective, the status and treatment of the elderly is more complex. Native Americans are a case in point. It is impossible to generalize about the Native American since tribes vary extensively in relation to customs, location, history, and acculturation. However, most values related to aging and the elderly among Native Americans are connected with having useful roles and being able to fulfill them (Schweitzer 1983).

In the past, older Native Americans' roles included caring for grandchildren and passing knowledge down to the young. Other roles were as midwives or healers, religious specialists, or social and political leaders. Power and prestige also was derived from patterns of land ownership and economic production that favored the old.

Today, the problems of older Native Americans parallel those of other minority or poor elderly. The loss of roles and of respect for elder knowledge, as the young move into the larger society and traditions are lost, has created a type of **anomie**, or loss of meaning, and the result for many has been isolation, alcoholism, disease, and despair (Kunitz 1983). Biomedical care for such conditions does not address their societal roots.

Biomedicine, Change, and the Elderly

The change from acute infectious disease to chronic degenerative diseases as a major cause of death in this century has been termed the "epidemiological revolution" and has major implications for health care. For many years, cultural attitudes about the elderly, as well as about growing old, were reflected in biomedicine, which viewed the needs and changes in capacities of the aging mind and body as simply inevitable and generally not matters for medical intervention. As people age, there is a greater need to make the patient feel comfortable, asking questions and voicing concerns in order to monitor intake of medications, capacities for self-care, and understanding of and agreement with treatment regimens for both patient and family. As the population ages, however, the role of medicine will be tied to culturally changing attitudes and to other institutions in determining quality, as much as quantity, of life for the elderly.

DEATH: THE FINAL STAGE OF MORTAL LIFE

Dying is not optional. But all cultures devise different ways to deal with it—complete with explanations, grieving procedures, celebration, and ritual. In Western culture, death has become institutionalized and hidden; the focus has shifted away from the dead to others' response to the demise of loved ones. Survivors attempt to hide emotions, the body is whisked off to the mortician's offices immediately, the coffin becomes a "casket," the body is embalmed to give the appearance of being life-like or natural, and mourning is carefully orchestrated to the visitation and funeral (Corr, Nabe, and Corr 1997: 71–72). The standardization of certain aspects of the modern rituals of death, such as disposal of the body, is now based upon public health concerns and therefore subject to law.

Over twenty years ago, Aries (1974) noted that the dying person is "deprived of his or her own death; mourning is denied; and new funerary rites are invented in the United States" (74). In the United States, over 80 percent of deaths now take place in the hospital, often alone, rather than in a domestic space surrounded by family and friends (Turner 1995: 126). Survivors rarely see the bodies of the dead except fleetingly. They generally do not touch them. These cultural practices send messages about core American values, such as the focus on sanitation, emotional control, and individuality.

Other conceptualizations, however, do exist. Like birth and other significant passages in the life course, dying and death are accompanied by a myriad of social and cultural meanings and rituals. Attending to traditions can be comforting and an essential part of the grieving process. It is important, therefore, as an expression of caring and respect, for health care workers confronted with death to encourage the dying and their survivors to attend to practices that are important to them.

Death in a Subculture

Asian Americans are an extremely diverse group with equally diverse cultural roots and customs. Their numbers are composed of Pacific Islanders and people of Chinese, Filipino, Japanese, and other origins. Although personal variations may be considerable, representing a large number of intervening variables, studies have found that grieving Japanese Americans tend to be quite restrained in expressing their feelings (Kalish and Reynolds 1981), and Chinese Americans tend to be "stoic" when facing death (Eisenbruch 1984). Many Asian Americans also tend not to directly question authority (Manio and Hall 1987), which can often lead to miscommunication and misconceptions when dealing with health care providers. Cultural tendencies such as these are best treated with understanding and sensitivity.

Galanti (1991: 49–50) describes the case of a young Vietnamese man who was found clinically dead after an accident. He was placed on a ventilator until the family could be notified. When the family arrived, they informed the physician that they wished to keep the man on life support until the "right time for him to die." They had consulted an astrologer who advised waiting. Within a week, they announced that he could die, and the ventilator was discontinued.

Astrology is taken very seriously by many Asians, as well as some other groups. Dying at the "proper time," notes Galanti, signifies good fortune for the descendants of the deceased. Otherwise, the children will suffer negative fates. In this case, the family had a chance to avert this outcome.

The physician and medical staff in this case were stunned by the incident and sought information through books on astrology and through Vietnamese co-workers. They realized that cultural beliefs and values are a very real part of people's lives. Although it is not always possible to honor those beliefs and values, concessions can often be made, and the remedy may be as simple as a screen for privacy or allowing for cultural rituals.

Death and Biomedicine

There is some speculation that a fear of or inability to deal with death leads some individuals into the field of biomedicine. The doctor becomes St. George (or Georgia, as the case may be), battling the enemy death, the dragon. When death occurs, however, it is often seen as failure on the part of the doctor.

Death has become medicalized and is managed and controlled by physicians, at least up to the point when a patient is defined as "dying" (Muller and Koenig 1988: 371). That particular point seems to be key in deter-mining the role and participation of physicians in the care of seriously ill (and perhaps dying) patients. Muller and Koenig (1988) found that medical interns tended not to define a patient as dying as long as there was some-thing (anything) to do (i.e., to treat), or the physician viewed (or con-structed) the patient as "having a chance." Once the patient has been defined as "dying," doctors may feel they have nothing more to do. They then tend to disappear, leaving the dying to nurses and family.

But the point at which a patient is defined as dying may not be the same point at which patient or family recognize that death is imminent. Patients (or their legal representatives) may decide to reject further treatment and ask to be allowed to die at home among friends and family or in a hospice setting. The hospice concept and philosophy, developed in England, centers around holistic care to the patient and family as a unit, and helping the patient live until s/he dies—*not* extending the dying process while the pa-tient lives. Care includes ongoing teamwork that is directed to the patient and family's various needs, including pain control with adequate doses of pain medication, withdrawal of active treatment, home care where possible, the provision of a humane and loving environment that affirms life and allows death, and continuing support of bereaved family after the death (Corr, Nabe, and Corr 1997: 199–200). This philosophy is notably in con-flict with the biomedical ideal of never giving up the fight for life and seeing death as failure.

As the technological possibilities change and multiply, more choices will have to be made. Social values, including the values of independent choice, family involvement, the value placed on "life," how life is to be defined, the weighing of economic priorities as well as supply versus demand, the consequences of medical intervention or no medical intervention—all must be considered in health care decision-making by clients as well as providers.

When biomedicine fails to meet our human and cultural needs, we may look elsewhere for care and support. In the following chapter, we examine other available systems that offer alternative or complementary modalities that, for various reasons, people may feel better suit their needs and ex-pectations.

FOR DISCUSSION

1. How does the life course affect the possibilities of health and illness in a population? How can awareness of life course issues be used in pro-viding health care?

2. What should be the role of the health care practitioner, including the physician, in dealing with personal and structural causal factors in illness

at each level of the life course? Why should the practitioner be concerned with nonbiomedical factors?

3. What changes have taken place in the life course that relate to health and illness or will most probably take place in the near future? How might they affect the delivery of health care?

4

Therapeutic Modalities: A Cross-Cultural Perspective

It is easy to make intellectual errors when dealing with medical systems. We forget that our own perspectives may prevent us from understanding the meaning and utility of practices that have been developed within another culture. That failure to account for our own needs and biases also can lead to the overenthusiastic acceptance of ideas whose genesis and application we really do not understand.

[Ergil 1996: 185]

Goal: To describe the diversity of ways in which humans view the body and its workings, conceptualize illness, and provide health care within different and sometimes overlapping systems.

Goal: To demonstrate that there are various approaches to healing and various categories of healers; to describe some of the key differences and similarities in both approaches and categories, and to show how different systems may be complementary.

When Jennifer began feeling lethargic and her occasional migraine headaches became more frequent, she thought perhaps it was just the stress of work. However, when her problems began to affect her work, a close friend recommended that she see a homeopath, Dr. Senseman, who had successfully treated him. Jennifer had never heard of homeopathy, but decided to give it a try. Dr. Senseman took a comprehensive history, allowing Jennifer to talk for over an hour, and then prescribed a remedy delivered in tiny white sugar pills. Within a week, Jennifer was feeling much better, and the headaches had not returned.

Jennifer's case reminds us that there are a multitude of ways we may perceive or respond to pain or illness. What is available to us and what we choose to do and why are inextricably bound up with our culture. The social structure allows or provides one or numerous alternatives, and our own socialization and perceptions provide our motivation for action. This chapter compares and contrasts the various ways that cultures influence us in perceiving illness and meeting our health needs.

Several scholars have created typologies that attempt to describe the range and use of various therapeutic systems or **modalities** and to highlight related cultural issues. Despite the best of intentions, most typologies are founded on ethnocentric assumptions, such as the primacy or superiority of one system over another. However, this is not in all cases a fatal flaw. We all have biases; the trick is to try to understand our biases and to anticipate how they may be reflected in thoughts and actions. As long as the assumptions in the frameworks we use to understand other people's choices are acknowledged, and the reasons for our adhering to them made clear, they may still facilitate our thinking about health issues.

Another problem with health typologies is that they are descriptive but generally not explanatory models. People using them may become so concerned with categorizing or naming things in accordance with the scheme at hand that they lose sight of the goal of understanding the various classified elements.

Further, classification schemes by definition fragment reality, carving it up into knowable chunks. This can camouflage the fact that the elements together might form a system, the whole of which is larger than the sum of the single parts that make it up. And schemes applied cross-culturally can be problematic because they ask us to evaluate cultural traits or items in a way that divorces them from their cultural context (cf. Augé and Herzlich 1995).

Finally, many health events or care approaches straddle the lines set forth in the classification schemes. In many cases, it is helpful to think of categories as having a continuum running between them.

HEALTH CARE CATEGORIES: THREE SCHEMES

The Three Medical Sectors of Kleinman

One typology commonly referred to is the **tripartite scheme** of popular, folk, and professional medicine first put forth by Arthur Kleinman (1986a [1978]). In this scheme, there are three sectors of health care, and the key variable is who provides care, in what context. **Popular** sector treatment is based on shared cultural understandings and is provided by nonspecialists, like one's self, one's mother, one's friends, or other kin and relations. **Folk** sector healers are specialists whose practice is based on traditional methods and philosophies. Legally sanctioned official systems (e.g., biomedical) make up what Kleinman called the **professional** sector.

When it was introduced twenty years ago, this typology was helpful as a starting point for thinking about medical care. It is an advance on simple "public-private" dichotomizing, in which private or household care is generally bounded as completely separate and is discounted. Kleinman's scheme allows for the interpenetration of these two arenas and values events that take place in the home. However, the division of labor by gender is not considered, which downplays the large contribution of women.

The terms chosen also are problematic. Although Kleinman (1986a [1978]) specifically allows that some nonbiomedical practices, such as Ayurvedic medicine (soon described) and chiropractic, should be classed as professional sector offerings due to their routinized, formalized, professionalized nature, this is easily forgotten by those who would view those therapeutic modalities as folk practices.

Perhaps more important, in some societies, no healing practices are professionalized and all are quite informal. As Gilbert Lewis explains, "There may be no separation of a department of knowledge and practice specifically orientated towards human sickness. Illness may be treated by religious or other specialists as one of their many duties; the explanations to account for it may stem from theories or premises that have much wider relevance than to sickness alone" (1986: 135). The notions of a distinct health system and of professionalization are somewhat culture-bound, limiting the universal applicability of Kleinman's tripartate scheme. Nonetheless, it is relevant to the current organization of health systems in the United States and other developed nations. But its relevance is hindered by the fact that the scheme has only three parts. There are many different types of healers in our folk and professional sectors, and a more elaborate scheme may be necessary if we are to fully understand the internal workings of these systems.

Wardwell's Typology: Relations with Biomedicine

A slightly more complex but biomedically centered scheme has been devised by Wardwell (1972). This typology categorizes various therapies according to similar basic characteristics. But therapies are also identified with respect to their relationship to the biomedical system, which is not per se listed as part of the typology. Thus the biomedical system serves as the yardstick for judging the social acceptability and different approaches of other systems of health care relative to biomedicine. The typology may be of use, however, in observing the directions and effects of social change on health care, and identifying the types and shifting relationships of various therapeutic modalities.

Wardwell classified practitioners other than physicians and nurses (who were termed **orthodox**), as limited, marginal, and quasi. **Limited** practitioners are independent of but accepted by the medical profession and treat particular areas of the human body; **marginal** practitioners generally treat a full range of disorders, but use therapies unacceptable to medical professionals. **Quasi**-practitioners are those whose therapies are pseudoscientific, nonmedical, and often incidental to another, possibly religious, function (250).

Limited practitioners include podiatrists, dentists, optometrists, and clinical psychologists. Pharmacists were included in the model as having a unique status—vis-à-vis physicians—which was labeled "ancillary." Having close public contact, pharmacists are often asked by clients to advise on remedies without physician intervention—a function objected to by physicians as an encroachment of their territory.

Marginal practitioners include chiropractors, homeopaths, naturopaths, reflexologists, acupuncturists, and formerly osteopaths, who have since moved into the biomedical sector. The key to the so-called marginality of these practitioners resides mostly in the fact that they tend to reject the biomedical approaches and support a monocausal theory of illness (e.g., chiropractors hold that the major cause of illness is misalignment of the spine). They also generally shun the use of drugs as poisons and often have a tradition of hostility toward biomedical practitioners.

The quasi-practitioners include those that remain—the faith healers, magical healers, and quacks. There are long traditions behind these healers, whose success is seen as mainly psychotherapeutic and, in the case of the quacks, exploitative. Any psychotherapeutic benefits, however, have generally not been recognized by the biomedical profession, which tends to see most of these systems as exploitative.

Christian Science is somewhat of a special case, stemming from the religious philosophy of Mary Baker Eddy, but unique in conceptual structure and therapies. Christian Scientists believe that matter, sin, pain, death, and sickness do not exist. All that is is spirit, God, and good. Healing, for Christian Scientists, generally involves resolving personal, social, and spiritual problems either alone or with the aid of a trained practitioner, through prayer and mental concentration (Wardwell 1972: 265).

Wardwell's typology can help us sort through various therapeutic modalities, even though it does not explain their varied popularity and appeal or costs and benefits. We would also revise the classification scheme somewhat to include biomedicine as one sector of the typology, based on the biomedical model of disease, and including physicians, nurses, psychiatrists, and so on; we would include an adjunct classification to include many of the more recently developed service providers such as emergency medical technicians, radiologists, x-ray technicians, physical therapists, respiratory therapists, and others whose functions are assistant to biomedicine.

With the use of a more balanced and expanded typology, it should be

Table 4.1
Medical Modalities: Some Key Typologies

Kleinman (1978)

Professional (e.g., biomedicine, Ayurveda)

Folk (e.g., faith healing)

Popular (e.g., mother's care)

Wardwell (1972) [our adapted version]

Biomedical (e.g., licensed to M.D.s; nurses)

Adjunct (e.g., medical technicians)

Limited (e.g., dentists)

Marginal (e.g., chiropractors)

Quasi-medical (e.g., faith healers; quacks)

Young (1983)

Accumulating (e.g., biomedicine, Ayurveda)

Diffusing (e.g., shamanism)

---

possible to discern other patterns, such as growth or decline and shortcomings and advantages of changing modalities. The typology can also be useful in tracking cross-referential complementary interactions (e.g., physicians who refer to chiropractors, chiropractors and physicians who practice homeopathy or acupuncture, faith healers and shamans who work with physicians, etc.). Examining this interaction can help us to identify the various dimensions of human need, complementarity, and the various outcomes when therapies are combined.

Young's Distinction: Accumulating and Diffusing Medicines

Allan Young (1983) recognized that biomedicine was not a universal yardstick for measuring all other systems. He divided all medical systems according to whether they entailed accumulated, formalized teachings or, rather, encouraged the fragmentation and diffusion of medical knowledge.

Accumulating and diffusing systems can be seen as on a continuum. **Accumulating** systems involve the collection of knowledge, generally in written form, conferences at which knowledge is shared, professional associations, and institutions for formal training. Biomedicine is an extreme version of an accumulating system. Chinese medicine, Ayurveda, Unani, and Galenic systems of medicine (all to be described) are also accumulating systems. **Diffusing** systems, on the other hand, do not have forums for communication between practitioners. Knowledge often is guarded as secret and rarely shared. Some shamans and magical healers working on their own are participants in diffusing systems (Young 1983: 1206). While this typology is limited by its simplicity, it demonstrates how looking at medicine from a different angle can open up new options for cross-cultural comparisons.

ANATOMY AND PHYSIOLOGY CROSS-CULTURALLY

Our conceptions about medical modalities aren't the only understandings we draw on in relation to health. When we try to fix something or to maintain it in good working order, many of our actions are guided by the way in which we think it has been put together. Health cultures everywhere entail ideas about how the body works. While cross-cultural differences in these ideas are vast, bodies themselves are generally the same worldwide, and there are many underlying similarities in different people's anatomical and physiological notions. Further, as women provide the majority of primary care, many basic ideas about the body may be gynocentric, or modeled on female caretakers' own bodies' functioning (Sobo 1993).

Not only do we share, as human beings, the same basic body form and structure worldwide, but we also live under the same laws of physics. Rivers blocked by logs or debris overflow their banks; rust stiffens or petrifies hinges; heat melts ice or causes other solids to soften, and cold temperatures cause liquids to coagulate. While the material aspect of these processes will differ cross-culturally (e.g., for the Eskimo the melting item might be snow; for the West Indian without a freezer it might be asphalt or fruit softening in the sun), the basic principles evinced will be the same. The basic principles also provide a framework for metaphorical elaboration. Many aspects of cross-cultural understandings about the body are simply elaborate abstractions of these basic principles, or selective but honest descriptions of basic, universal, embodied experiences (Lakoff 1987; M. Johnson 1987).

Human beings are creative. In addition to building on basic-level models to create explanatory systems, people exposed to different technologies will use different metaphors from these technologies to describe and understand body functions. Emily Martin demonstrates this in relation to the historical changes our own society has undergone: with industrialization, the body was increasingly imaged as a factory, converting energy into products (1987: 36–37). Importantly, like the factory—indeed like our society in general (government provides a good illustration)—the body was seen as hierarchically organized rather than as made up of systems that functioned as a committee of equals, each exerting mutual influence. Body and society are, in many ways, **homologous** (equivalent; literally, having the same structure).

The Inner Body

Many people worldwide have not spent much time exploring the inner cavities of the body. But experience tells us that the torso contains at least one large cavity. Sometimes, there are a number of large cavities connected by pipes or tubes. Jamaicans, for example, view the trunk as divided into two spaces: the chest, and the belly, which extends from just under the breast to the groin. Almost 60 percent of the participants in a British study also viewed the belly as such (Boyle 1970, as cited in Helman 1995: 18–19).

Societies that slaughter animals for food and so regularly have direct dealings with their viscerae (or who have ancestors who did) might envisage the cavities as full of sacs or bags. Jamaicans do: The belly, for example, holds air sacs (lungs), a urine bag (bladder), and, in women, a baby bag (womb).

Flow, Blockage, and Cleanliness

Elaborations on a basic spatial, hydraulic model that emphasizes flow and balance and incorporates container and conduit imagery (which Sobo [1993] calls a "flow model") can be found in ethnographic descriptions of a range of cultures (e.g., Laguerre 1987; Snow 1993). They are commonly invoked in lay explanations of menstruation (Buckley and Gottlieb 1988; Sobo 1992); they are also a common and important part of indigenous theories of contraception or abortion and fertility enhancement (e.g., Browner 1985; Ngin 1985; Nichter and Nichter 1987; Shedlin 1982). Flow models are described for the Amazonian Mehinaku (Gregor 1985: ch. 5), the Hua of New Guinea (Meigs 1983), and for biomedical scientists (Martin 1987: ch. 3). Mexican ideas about *empacho*, in which digestion is blocked and food adheres to intestines or the stomach wall where it grows moldy, also indicate a flow model (Young and Garro 1982: 1459; Stafford 1978: 16).

In a flow system, it is essential that nothing block the body's pipes or tubes. To ensure that this does not happen, and for alleviation if it does, people can take occasional purges, as with laxatives. If left unattended, waste can build up behind blockages and fester, turning septic; blockages themselves can rot, releasing toxins into the system. In the United Kingdom, many fear what Helman calls "the dangers of constipation," which include the release of impurities into the bloodstream (1995: 25). Lynn Payer reports that some refer to this process as "autointoxication" (1989: 116). These theories and beliefs help to explain the therapies adopted, which include treatments such as purging with enemas or medicines to reestablish or maintain flow. Even if such therapy does not make biomedical sense (and sometimes it does) it makes cultural sense, following a logic for which culture provides the basis.

Purges in many cultures are meant to cleanse all bodily systems, including the circulatory system, urinary system, and respiratory system. The medicines that affect these internal cleanings can, but need not be, specialized;

for many, bodily systems are interconnected and drainage is through the bottom parts, so waste from all of them might be excreted out in feces or flushed out on urination. Similarly, vomiting (whether induced or naturally occurring) might serve this purpose.

Likewise, poisons may be drawn out through the skin, as with poultices (facial masks, popular with some American women, work this way) or through cupping or coin rubbing. The latter therapy, associated with Asian cultures, involves rubbing a coin on the skin to "draw out" the illness. In cupping, a heated cup is placed on the skin, creating a vacuum. As with coin rubbing, cupping can leave raised red welts.

People often use coin rubbing on children. The welts might suggest intentional child abuse. It is essential to realize that this is not the case, but that coin rubbing is done as a demonstration of love and caring (Korbin 1987: 28).

KATHY NGUYEN

A Vietnamese girl named Kathy Nguyen was in her first year at an American elementary school. She was not feeling very well one morning so her mother rubbed the back of her neck with a coin. She then felt well enough to attend school. Later in the day, however, she began to feel worse and went to see the school nurse. When the nurse discovered the welts on Kathy's neck, she immediately assumed she was seeing a case of child abuse and conscientiously reported the Nguyens to the authorities. The situation was finally straightened out, but it created a great deal of needless embarrassment and stress for Kathy's family. (Galanti 1991: 96)

KEEPING EQUILIBRIUM

Not all cultures are so focused on keeping the internal body clean or flow unimpeded. But most do have some notion of equilibrium, and strive to maintain some sort of balance (cf. Young 1986 [1976]: 140–41) For example, in Vermont, people have used honey and vinegar (acid and alkali) to help maintain bodily balance (Atkinson 1978: 175). Biomedical practitioners themselves talk often of balance: hormone imbalances, vitamin deficiencies, bacterial imbalances in the gut, and many other problems are conceptualized in terms of an equilibrium model of health.

Hot and Cold

In many Latin American and Caribbean cultures, and in some others, maintaining a balance between hot and cold is essential. Illness happens when the body (which generally is self-regulating) becomes too cool or too hot. For instance, among many Latin Americans and Caribbeans, menstruation and childbirth both are hot states. The body heats up and expels either menstrual blood or a baby. A hot body is open or vulnerable to the penetration of cold and other forces in a way that the body ordinarily would not be. Dangerous exposure must be avoided.

To this end, postpartum Puerto Ricans in one U.S. study reported avoiding cold foods. Ingestion of such foods would lead their postpartum discharges to clot and solidify, perhaps leading the waste in the discharge to be reabsorbed into the body rather than running out. This could cause nervousness or madness. To offset this threat, the women drank tonics containing garlic, chocolate, cinnamon, and other foods classified as hot (Snow and Johnson 1978).

In some contexts, rather than to counterbalance disequilibrium, treatments seek to further heat or cool the body. For example, if the body is heating up in order to expel some toxin, further heating might help the body accomplish this task, thereby speeding recovery.

Importantly, although sick bodies do feel hot and cold, hot and cold are not necessarily thermal designations but rather symbolic constructions concerning the essential character of an item or state. Classification may be based on color (or darkness or lightness), gender associations (maleness or femaleness), origin (e.g., foods from the sea or grown underground are cold while foods grown in direct sunlight are hot), and nutritive value (often, foods seen as supernutritious are hot) (Logan 1977: 490). Sometimes the designation of a food, substance, or act as hot or cold is an after-the-fact justification of empirically observed bodily effects (Foster 1994: 75).

Body Fluids

Sometimes, thermal systems are balanced around not only heat and coolness, but also dryness and wetness, and specific body fluids can be involved. In French medicine, the liver and its bile are central (Payer 1989). In African Caribbean, as well as in African American medicine, blood is key.

Jill Korbin and Maxene Johnston (1982) describe a conflict over blood testing in a pediatric hospital that pitted a mother from Belize against a staff of biomedical clinicians. The mother felt that clinicians were harming her sick daughter with diagnostic blood tests, which she felt were needless. She was concerned about the loss of blood and the disequilibrium in her small daughter's already weak body that was bound to happen if blood drawing did not stop. Accused of ignorance and child abuse, and threatened with legal action, the mother resorted to bringing her daughter herbal teas to " 'build her blood back up' " (261). It is worth mentioning that in addition to her worries about blood depletion, the mother feared that hospital staff members were drawing excess quantities of blood so that they could sell it for a profit.

Sometimes, when people use the word "blood," they refer to something altogether different, and this issue is quite relevant in the context of health care provision. For Caribbean peoples, for example, blood comes in two types: white and red. When unqualified by adjective or context, the word "blood" in Jamaica means the red kind, built from thick, dark liquid items such as red bean soup, English-style stout, or red-colored edibles such as tomatoes.

"*Sinews*," another form of blood, comes from okra, fish eyes, and other light-colored gelatinous foods, such as egg whites. Overexposure to the sun or excess tiring work can dry it out. Sinews include, but is not limited to, synovial fluid, which does resemble egg whites and lubricates the joints. The eyes are filled with sinews and glide in their sockets with its aid. Sinews is also associated with the nerves and with procreation. Many call it "white" blood in comparison to the red. Both kinds of blood are essential for good health.

Because the blood is so important, its qualities must be monitored. Not only must it be kept clean and thermally regulated, but it also must be neither too thick nor too thin, too bitter nor too sweet, too high nor too low in the body.

Balance in Accumulating Systems

Worldwide, a number of societies have developed highly sophisticated equilibrium-based accumulating systems of health by elaborating on the basic idea of bodily balance so that many body components and many types of qualities are implicated. These systems, generically called **humoral systems** because they all involve humors or body substances, refer not only to the physiological workings of the human body, but also to social interactions and to cosmological concepts and nonorganic elements as well. As Charles Leslie writes, "The arrangement and balance of elements in the human body were microcosmic versions of their arrangement in society at large and throughout the universe" (1976: 4). Factors such as sex, age, the season, diet, activities, and the tenor of one's relationships influence a person's equilibrium.

Classic humoral medicine, or Galenic medicine, stems from Hippocratic medicine (after the Greek theorist Hippocrates, 460 B.C.). The Greek physician Galen systematized and adapted the Hippocratic teachings into the Galenic system, which dominated in Europe until the germ theory of the late 1900s changed the direction of scientific medical investigation (Magner 1992: 93).

Galenic medicine teaches that the body contains four liquids or humors: blood, phlegm (mucus), yellow bile (stomach secretions, as in vomit), and black bile (according to Foster, possibly fecal matter darkened by blood; 1994: 5). Each humor has hot or cold and wet or dry properties, and each is associated with a "complexion" or temperament: sanguine (ruddy, cheerful), phlegmatic (lethargic), bilious (ill-tempered), and melancholic (sad). Further associations were made between humors and basic elements (accordingly, four were identified: wind or air, water, fire, and earth), as well as with the four seasons. As long as the four humors are in balance, health ensues. Imbalance can be treated by removing excesses, as by purging or vomiting, or by correcting for deficiencies that can be made up through special diets.

Knowledge of Galenic medicine gradually diffused eastward. The system diffused was called Tibb-i-Yunani in Arabic, or Unani, which means Greek medicine (Foster 1994: 13; Leslie 1976: 2). Today, many Islamic people maintain hot-cold distinctions, base their diet on Unanic precepts, and even divide all drugs according to these qualities (Nasr 1968: 228).

At the end of the seventh century, Moslems were moving westward, and Galenic medicine diffused to Spain and Portugal via northern Africa and then to Latin America (Foster 1994: 14). Foster argues that the most important roots of thermal equilibrium systems in Latin America stem from Europe. However, the universal experiential basis of hot-cold conceptualizations and notions of balance suggest that equilibrium models would have existed in Latin America and the Caribbean, even without colonialism, as locally generated variations on a universal theme. European knowledge was incorporated if suitable and useful and was rejected if not.

Some Galenic teachings also were taken into the Ayurvedic system, a similarly complex system that dates back some 4,000 years and is now practiced mainly in North India, but also in Pakistan, Bangladesh, Sri Lanka, and throughout the Arab world (Gesler 1991: 16). In Ayurveda, there are only three humors (phlegm, bile, and wind or flatulence), but there are seven body components: blood, flesh, fat, bone, marrow, semen, and food juice. Five elements exist: ether, which is like the atmosphere, is the fifth. As in Greek medicine, heat and coolness also are important, and balance ensures good health (Foster 1994: 8).

The same is true in traditional Chinese medicine. However, this system centers on two contrasting forces: *yin* and *yang*. Yin subsumes all that is dark, moist, watery, and female; yang is comprised of all that is light, dry, fiery, and male. The idea of specific humors—and in Chinese medicine there are six (Leslie 1976: 4)—seems to have been appended to an initial yin-yang matrix (Foster 1994: 11). In any case, each organ is associated with yin or yang, and sophisticated procedures such as acupuncture, whereby needles are inserted into particular spots on the body and manipulated, are used to free up or redirect the energy flow. A basic concept of this system is that of the vital life force, or *qi*. Each individual body is pervaded by this energy, which allows physical function and maintains health and vitality (Ergil 1996: 195).

Chinese medicine, used as early as 1500 B.C., is still practiced in China, which for around three decades has had an extensive national program of combining traditional and Western medicine as formal components of their health care system (Bodeker 1996: 281). It is also practiced in Chinese communities throughout the world.

Kleinman (1984) observed that despite their relative independence, there have been various degrees of borrowing and modernization in all these systems; he sees this as "a sign of a living, changing tradition in contradistinction to an historical artifact" (148). That is, these traditions, like any traditions, are not monolithic and unitary, but are constantly undergoing change, as is biomedicine.

Leslie reminds us, however, that these traditions "maintained their individual characters although they were in contact with each other. The integrity of the separate traditions needs to be emphasized" (1976: 2). And although they were "relatively independent," these health traditions "evolved in similar ways," all becoming professional branches of scientific learning with professional standards for education and practice (3).

As with the biomedical profession, authority of practitioners in these accumulating systems is vested in highly respected texts, special ways of dressing, and ethical codes (Leslie 1976: 3). The theoretical bases for these systems were also derived by the "scientific method" if we understand by that term logical reasoning and conclusions based upon observations of various phenomena. The concepts of balance, flow, energy, temperature, and so forth, are not so foreign to biomedicine: after all, blood pressure readings measure blood flow; specialists talk of one's hormonal or electrolyte balance; thermoregulation is at stake in conditions like hypothermia; and fevers, measured with thermometers, indicate infections.

Body Size and Shape

Body concepts are not limited to physiology. Cultures also have ideals for body shape and size. One area that has lately received much attention is weight, reflecting our own culturally constructed concern over fatness. In her cross-cultural review on the topic, Cassidy (1991) found that socially dominant individuals with sound relationships are usually large (relatively speaking). Bigness tends to ensure reproductive success and survival in times of scarcity and, cross-culturally, plumpness is generally considered attractive.

Such is the case in many of the West African societies from which people were taken to the United States as slaves. In some of these societies, those who can afford to do so seclude their adolescent girls in special "fattening rooms" and, after a period of ritual education and heavy eating, the girls emerge fat, attractive, and nubile (Brink 1989).

In Jamaica, as in other Caribbean societies where a respected adult is called a "big man" or a "big woman," good relations involve food-sharing, and people on good terms with others are (ideally) large. Weight loss signals social neglect. A Jamaican seeing someone grow thin wonders about the sorts of life stresses that have caused the weight loss, rather than offering congratulations for it and attributing it to a "good" diet, as many middle- and upper-class Americans do. U.S. residents living in our inner cities, on the other hand, also worry about weight loss among friends or relatives. Thinness might be a symptom of HIV infection or tuberculosis, it may indicate that a person is addicted to crack cocaine or other dangerous substances, or it may simply signify poverty.

In the United States, being plump (i.e., categorized as overweight) is generally associated with unattractiveness, especially in females, and this has been connected with the rise in eating disorders—specifically anorexia nervosa and bulimia. Plumpness itself may be seen as signifying "moral laxity" or a lack of self-control, which may lead to discrimination in employment (Bordo 1993; Wolf 1991: 179–217).

Sexual Biology: An Objective Science?

The conceptualization of male and female bodies also differs from society to society—geographically as well as historically. For example, while mainstream medicine presently views male and female bodies as two distinct entities, Thomas Laqueur (1990) has shown that sexual difference was, until recently, a matter of degree and not kind among many Europeans. "Language marks this view of sexual difference," he says. "For two millennia the ovary, an organ that by the early nineteenth century had become a synecdoche for woman, had not even a name of its own. Galen refers to it with the same word he uses for the male testes"(4-5); a synecdoche is a metaphor in which a part (ovary) stands for a whole (woman). Because men and women were viewed as more similar than distinct prior to the latter 1700s, male genitalia could be understood as merely the external expression of what in females was retained in the internal area of the groin. The penis, for example, was understood as an extruded vagina (Laqueur 1990).

But for various reasons, in the eighteenth century, a belief in fundamental differences replaced the belief in congruity between the sexes. This led anatomists to focus not on similarities, but on distinctions between the male and female body. A vast amount of data demonstrating no difference between male and female anatomy and physiology, such as the fact that male and female reproductive organs share common developmental origins from the fetal stage, was ignored or treated as if absent while differences in form and function were highlighted.

Biology is not, then, so objective. The body is not the unmovable ground that we like to think it is. Culture determines, to some degree, the size and shape we see as natural, and what we find when we peer inside the body. What explains the cultural shift in ways of seeing the body that led from the one-sex to the two-sex model? As Laqueur explains, after the French Revolution, custom lost its force: the new egalitarianism threatened to undermine men's superordinate position. So the gender status quo was justified by grounding female inferiority and subordination in her distinct biological make-up. Biology became destiny. Laqueur (1990) thus demonstrates that biology and medicine are culturally influenced fields that can serve to underpin dominant ideologies. In the words of Allan Young, "medical practices are simultaneously ideological practices" (1982: 271).

Body, Mind, and Society

Health cultures are not concerned solely with the body corporeal (Frankenberg's term; 1994: 1326). They also entail ideas about the mind or the conscious, interactive self and ways to keep it in good order. Some of these concern good living—conducting oneself in keeping with the recommended social and moral order. For example, maintaining good interpersonal relations limits one's exposure to strong emotions, which might affect the mind, and to the wrath of others, which might be vented on one's health. Such relations may include those with kin, friends, and neighbors, as well as deceased relatives or other spiritual entities.

Improper treatment of the corporeal or physical body also can affect the mind, just as mind trouble can manifest itself in the corporeal body. In fact, these two dimensions of experience—mental and physical—are inextricably interconnected. Ailments centered in one dimension of the person will often have ramifications in the other. So treatment of the mind may involve treatment of the body, and vice versa.

For example, biomedical doctors may treat nervousness with medications designed to alter brain chemistry. Jamaicans also focus treatments for nervousness on the body, prescribing certain remedies and food supplements meant to strengthen the physical nerves and restore a certain kind of "white" blood, the lack of which contributes to nerve problems (Sobo 1996b).

But in certain Latin American cultures, the symptoms of nerves may be attributed ultimately to soul loss (literally, loss of the soul), and ritual as well as physical action will need to be taken. The physical processes immediately underlying a condition, sometimes called the immediate or **proximate cause**, is not as important as the **ultimate cause**—the reason why that problem is bothering that individual at that point in time. Indeed, physical processes might not even be implicated at all in particular forms of suffering or distress. This demonstrates the necessity of a broad conceptualization of health; most health systems worldwide involve and address far more than simple physical problems when restoring or promoting good health.

SEEKING HEALTH

Recognizing Symptoms

It is quite possible to be ill without being diseased. Likewise, it is possible to have a disease without being ill. Illness is not merely a person's reaction to a disease. Indeed, it is not disease that spurs a person to seek medical treatment, but rather, as Robert Hahn points out, it is his or her "experience of suffering which engenders the whole medical enterprise. The sufferer's judgment rather than that of biomedicine defines the *underlying problem*" (1984: 17; emphasis in original; also see Mechanic 1962).

The underlying problem, or sickness, according to Hahn, "is a matter of unwanted conditions of self" (1995: 22). And while certain conditions will be universally unwanted, "what is major sickness for one may be a minor irritation for another" (23); a sore knee will merely bother the academic but will be cause for great alarm in the Olympic athlete. Unwanted conditions of self not only vary from individual to individual but also from culture to culture: "the good Buddhist pursues experiences of generalized hopelessness for which the Westerner seeks treatment" (Hahn 1995: 35).

The recognition of symptoms, the first step in what Noel Chrisman terms "the health seeking process," depends on cultural definitions of normal health, as well as understandings about the causes and contexts of sickness (1977). Some of the important factors here are symptom visibility and frequency. The visibility and frequency of the symptom in question in others and the way this compares to its visibility and frequency in one's own case is key, for the former provides a context for evaluating the significance of the latter. Also taken into account is the level of danger to life and interference with lifestyle, or disability, that the symptoms or the syndrome entailed portend.

Chrisman's inclusion of the degree to which the individual thinks that something can be done is also a part of the Health Belief Model (HBM), a theoretical framework for predicting the likelihood for care-seeking (Rosenstock 1966; also see Becker 1974). This model posits that an individual's subjective evaluation of an illness situation, including the value placed on a particular outcome and the belief that a particular action will result in that outcome, becomes the key variable in the utilization of health services. The patient's "common sense" may conflict with clinical judgment (see Becker and Maiman 1975).

In addition to being self-defined, ill-health can be other-defined, in which case others perceive an individual's symptoms, define them as an illness condition, and then call the illness to the individual's attention (Mechanic 1978). Although the biomedical system is organized so that individual patients present their own cases, in reality many people are assisted by others when it comes to identifying and interpreting symptoms and weighing treatment options.

In any case, once symptoms are recognized, individuals may adopt a culturally prescribed **sick role**. The sick role, a concept introduced by Talcott Parsons, legitimizes sickness under four conditions: the individual who is sick is exempt from "normal" social roles, is not at fault or responsible for the sickness condition, should try to get well, and should seek technically competent help and cooperate with the physician (1951). Thus the physician becomes an agent of social control, and help-seeking elsewhere is not "legitimate."

The narrow bounds of legitimacy in this model, its middle-class orientation, postulations of role exemption and individual responsibility, definition of "technically competent help," and failure to address the variability of individuals and social groups have been criticized as biomedically biased and culturally limiting (Mechanic 1962; Gordon 1966; Twaddle 1969). However, the concept of the sick role does contribute to an understanding of the desirability of health for any culture, however defined. In addition, since many types of deviant behavior such as overeating, drug addiction, and smoking can endanger the public's health, medicine acts as an agent of social control under the auspices of the state. The sick role thus contributes to an understanding of the mechanisms of social stability (Turner 1984).

There are numerous other explanatory models and theories of illness perception (e.g., Suchman 1965; Freidson 1970), most of which have a number of similarities to those we have presented (i.e., Chrisman 1977; Hahn 1984, 1995; Mechanic 1978; Parsons 1951). All have some limitations; for example, many assume the goal of biomedical care as the legitimate response. But there are many other paths to health. Nonbiomedical approaches, those termed "complementary" or "alternative," are commonly used.

Complementary or Alternative Options

"**Complementary**" and "**alternative**" can be interchangeable terms. Micozzi, commenting on various definitions of the terms, explains them as generally referring to practices that are neither routinely taught in U.S. medical schools nor paid for by regular health insurance policies. However, the claim that alternative medicine is not a part of the existing health care system is curious in view of the millions of Americans who use alternative approaches after defining themselves as ill (1996a: 5).

It is problematic that the bulk of health-seeking theories basically relate to perception of symptoms and the consequent decision to visit a physician. Symptoms are not always grouped together in the same way cross-culturally, and the physician is not always the first or even last choice of provider. It is important for clinicians to ascertain why clients choose to consult them, to know exactly what clients think their symptoms mean, and to discuss their own inferences before prescribing a treatment regimen.

Also relevant here is the fact that many people who are diseased do not perceive themselves as ill, and vice versa. Since in most instances disease is self-limiting (e.g., a bout of flu generally ends even without medical treatment; cf. Kleinman 1986a [1978]: 33), this is not necessarily a bad thing. However, it may pose a problem for biomedical treatment regimens when no disease is found, and a problem for society when those who are sick get sicker or pass their disease to others. Understanding the cultural aspects of illness perception can therefore aid in protecting both individuals and society.

Patterns of Resort

Even in the United States, only 10 to 30 percent of medical problems are ever brought to the attention of a biomedical clinician (Zola, cited in Demers et al. 1980). In a 1980 study by Demers and colleagues, the figure was less than 6 percent. Despite the fact that all participants were covered for free biomedical treatments by prepaid medical insurance, most care was procured within the household. In one of four cases (24.7 percent), no action was taken. In slightly more than one in four cases (28.9 percent), home remedies were used. More often (38.7 percent), people self-medicated with over-the-counter preparations or prescription drugs left over from another occasion (1088).

Little research addresses the choice and use of diverse systems within the context of industrialized, biomedically dominated nations. An exception is the work of psychologists Furnham and Beard (1995), which focuses on patients' choice of complementary medicine over biomedicine. It seems that people visit complementary medical practitioners, or CMs, for reasons other than dissatisfaction with professional medicine. The most significant factor associated with visiting CM practitioners was health beliefs: people who visited CM practitioners believed more strongly that mental, emotional, and environmental factors play a significant part in both health and illness. These people also tended to emphasize the importance of positive attitudes and happiness and took more control of their own health behavior (e.g., self-medication). Further, they did not tend to "blame the victims" for their own fate. But it remains unclear whether health beliefs lead to choice of practitioner, or practitioners educate or lead clients to particular health beliefs; Furnham and Beard conclude it is probably a bit of both (1431).

The study did reveal that people may visit both a CM and biomedical practitioner at the same time, as well as using one or the other for specific problems. The different systems thus may become complementary in a very literal sense. An individual can also harbor both externally and internally oriented beliefs about causes of illness, not necessarily just one or the other. Personality factors appeared to be negligible. The study suggests that medical choice-making is a fertile field for research.

Multiple Treatment Modes

The concept of the biomedically oriented "lay-referral" system originated with Eliot Freidson (1960), who suggested that when people become ill, they first turn to family and friends, then to suggested lay "experts," and finally, if nothing works, to a physician and the biomedical system, although lay norms may influence this option. This behavior is consistent with Romanucci-Ross' "hierarchy of resort" (1969). However, while Romanucci-Ross was concerned with acculturation issues, most scholars who use the phrase today generally mean that people try the most familiar or simplest and cheapest treatment first and then seek more expensive, complex, or unfamiliar treatments if necessary.

While treatment choice can follow a hierarchical sequence, often patterns of resort are cumulative and quite pluralistic, involving many treatment modalities at once. And people do not necessarily comply with all the rules surrounding each type of treatment. People often creatively combine recommendations, coming up with the regimen they feel is right for them. As Chrisman (1977) has pointed out, the "health seeking process" is dynamic, and people are constantly reevaluating their symptoms and actions and revising their plans.

In many cases, people who seek biomedical assistance already have used some type of home treatment. Snow cites a Michigan study in which 78 percent of fifty elderly individuals being treated biomedically for hypertension had used home remedies in the past six months. When asked if their doctors knew, 80 percent said that they did not (1993: 128–29). A national study reported home remedy use frequency of 72 percent, and found that 89 percent of those using other therapies did so without their doctors' recommendation or knowledge (Eisenberg et al. 1993: 249).

In a representative nationwide telephone survey of adults, Eisenberg and colleagues (1993) found that one in three people have used at least one "unconventional" (nonbiomedical) therapy in the past year. One-third of these people saw providers for this therapy (rather than self-administering). The latter group made an average of nineteen visits during the last year, and these visits cost, on average, $27.60 each. Expenditure in 1990 amounted to about $13.7 billion, and three-quarters of this was paid out of pocket. These fees do not include the costs of drugs, such as herbals, or books or other healing materials. The number of visits, 425 million, exceeded the 388 million visits to all primary care physicians in 1990. These findings quite surprised the researchers. The study found no significant differences according to insurance status or to sex. However, significantly more people aged 25–49 used unconventional therapies than those who were older or younger.

Importantly, the term "unconventional therapy" used in this study covered many relatively expensive therapies that people cannot carry out at home, such as chiropractic and acupuncture, in addition to herbal medicine and such. In regard to home remedies in particular, however, it may be that more Blacks than Whites, as well as more older individuals and financially less well-off people, are more likely to use them. In her review, Snow noted that black men in Detroit were six times more likely than white men to use a home remedy; black women were three times more likely to do so than were white women (1993: 129).

THE MODALITIES: ETIOLOGICAL UNDERPINNINGS

Theoretical Frameworks of Various Systems

As Kavanagh and Kennedy note, "The common commodity among health-related disciplines is care" (1992: 21). Various therapeutic systems or modalities, aim to provide care, including healing, but they do so in different ways and with different aims, as different systems entail different definitions of what the well person looks and feels like and how that person is to be treated.

As diverse as medical systems are, there are many similarities cross-culturally. For example, the Pennsylvania Dutch, who have descended from German immigrants who settled in various areas of Pennsylvania, generally rely on **homeopathic** treatments. In homeopathy, the remedy, if used on a healthy person, would produce the same symptoms as those exhibited by the sick individual. This is not a unique concept; it is also used biomedically in treating allergies and in using live or dead viruses in minute amounts to stimulate the body's immune reactions.

In diagnosing and treating illness, it is sometimes important to know how the body normally functions and how, in sickness, those processes have been physiologically impeded. At other times, mental and social processes are deemed more important for isolating causes and devising treatment strategies than are physiological processes. Family therapists, for example, treat whole family units as systems that may have encouraged the presence of sickness (e.g., anorexia, alcoholism) in one member. Families are then taught to think in new ways, and to adopt different social interactions. Similarly, some shamans or diviners might treat illness by prescribing a confession and atonement session in which family members confess or declare wrongdoings to others and try to set their relationships right.

The latter type of treatment, which centers on social relations, is called "personalistic"; a modality in which individual biological pathologies are treated is called "naturalistic." Naturalistic treatment also can be addressed to illness brought about by strong emotions when these induce an internal, impersonal imbalance in the body. The **naturalistic-personalistic** scheme, which we discuss in more detail below, was offered by George Foster in the context of a cross-cultural examination of disease etiologies (theories of disease origins) in 1976. It does not take structural factors into account.

Another simple, two-part (and likewise structurally naive) etiological model holds that illness can stem from the bodily intrusion or extrusion of substances, essences, or objects. The **intrusion-extrusion** model we describe is adapted from and builds on early classification schemes such as that of Forrest Clements (1932). Extrusion-caused illness can occur as a result of soul loss or the loss of blood or nonabsorption of nutrients, as with diarrhea. In intrusion-caused illnesses, noxious substances such as poisons, germs, or evil spirits penetrate the body's barriers, disturbing its internal balance. In this model, illness due to a bleeding wound or to the loss of one's soul are classed together, just as germs and evil spirits are similarly categorized as intrusive. However, treatment for germ-caused or spirit-caused illness does differ, and this is what Foster was getting at with his 1976 naturalistic-personalistic typology.

Allan Young, also in 1976, described another two-part scheme in which illness was seen either as **internalized** or **externalized**. Internalizing systems, says Young, focus on physiological explanations or mechanisms, and on the "biophysical signs which mark the course of disease episodes" (1986 [1976]: 140). Illness is encapsulated in the individual body. Biomedicine would be a good example of an internalizing system.

Externalizing systems, on the other hand, ascribe more importance to events that happen outside of the body that is sick. In these systems, "pathogenic agencies are usually purposive and often human or anthropomorphized [i.e., conceptualized in human form]. Diagnostic interests concentrate on discovering what events could have brought the sick person to the attention of the pathogenic agency" (Young 1986 [1976]: 141). Externalizing systems are more concerned with ultimate causes than with proximate internal mechanisms. The Navajo practice of having a specialist sing, bringing the ill person's world back into balance, and thereby treating the root of his or her disorder, is part of an externalizing system (Adair, Deuschle, and Barnett 1988: 7, 170).

While there are subtle differences between the two schemes, the naturalistic-personalistic and internalizing-externalizing schemes in many ways overlap. Whether one or the other is invoked depends on the aspects of illness that the theorist seeks to highlight or explain.

Social Complexity, Cultural Unity, and Changing Medical Systems

Young (1986 [1976]) offers some important suggestions about the evolution of health systems using the externalizing-internalizing model that are worth mentioning. Young holds that internalizing systems evolved from externalizing systems in societies that grew complex, as happened in the United States with modernization and industrialization.

Externalizing systems focus on social and cosmological relations. They are interlinked with other cultural domains, such as religion. As Young says, externalizing systems have a "low degree of conceptual autonomy" (1986 [1976]: 143).

But internalizing systems are autonomous to a high degree. That is, physical health is not overtly linked to social or moral health. Young explains this as stemming from a division of labor. In small-scale societies, the division of labor is low, and there is not much specialization; according to Young (1986 [1976]) this explains the overlap between healing and other cultural domains (e.g., legal, religious, etc.).

As Peter Morley has commented, "The cognitive world of traditional societies tends to be less compartmentalized than that of the modern Western world. One aspect of life is usually inextricably intertwined with many others, not only situationally, but in the thought of those who inhabit technologically less developed societies" (1978: 2). Cecil Helman also has pointed out that beliefs about the causes of ill health often connect with beliefs about a wide range of types of misfortune, such as interpersonal conflicts, earthquakes, crop failures, theft, and other forms of loss (1995: 7).

In large-scale societies, we find complex patterns of labor division. The conceptual autonomy of internalizing schemes is, Young (1986 [1976]) says, linked to the emergence of specialization and extreme distinction between cultural domains, which comes with such complex patterns. In large-scale societies, where cultural realms are fragmented, internalizing medicines, which focus on the body and pay little attention to legal, religious, and other dimensions of life, can evolve.

In biomedicine, as in all internalizing systems, religion and magic have limited explanatory power; curers need no supernatural abilities. Health is segmented off from other aspects of culture, such as religion and social relationships (although, as chapter 3 showed, this is changing). Biomedicine even divorces mind from body, with different branches specializing in physical or mental health.

Naturalistic Approaches

While the externalizing-internalizing scheme is, in some contexts, quite useful, we find the naturalistic-personalistic model has more immediate or practical utility. The rest of the chapter examines the model in detail, and uses it to organize the presentation of practitioner types.

Naturalistic models explain sickness as being due to impersonal forces or conditions, including "cold, heat, winds, dampness, and, above all, by an upset in the balance of the basic body elements" (Foster 1976: 775).

Table 4.2
Practitioners

Naturalistic Practitioners	Personalistic Practitioners	
	Magical	*Religious*
Herbalists	Healers	Priests
Chemists	Sorcerers	Shamans
Surgeons		
Bodyworkers		
Midwives		

Foster explains that all naturalistic modalities are based on ideas of equilibrium. The humoral systems described earlier in this chapter are good examples, and so is biomedicine, which views illness as a disruption of function at a physiological level, whose causes may include attack by viruses and bacteria, breakdown of biological systems, and so on. Viewed naturalistically, illness can be treated without social, supernatural, or spiritual intervention.

Cross-culturally, five types of naturalistic practitioners exist: herbalists, chemists, surgeons, bodyworkers, and lay midwives (we will use the term "midwife" to indicate lay midwives, as opposed to midwives in the nursing profession). The inclusion of the midwife may seem strange because this category of healer is determined by the body system or event attended to, rather than by a method of healing per se (e.g., with herbs, or chemicals, or by cutting, or manipulating). Moreover, pregnancy is generally not defined cross-culturally as an illness to be healed; it was not considered so historically (see Eastman and Loustaunau 1987). Indeed, in various states, including New Mexico, midwives were not categorized as health care providers and thus were not subject to medical licensure until the 1920s. But midwifery is an extremely common occupation cross-culturally, with the purpose of providing care and assistance to preserve the health of the mother, and so we include it in our list (see Table 4.2).

The skills categories described here are not mutually exclusive; while in some cultures practitioners are extremely specialized, in others there may be a significant amount of overlap. Humoral doctors, for example, may be both chemists and herbalists. There may also be overlap in medical systems themselves; for example, biomedical and Ayurvedic approaches are used in combination by many practitioners in India where medical **syncretism**, or the active aggregation or blending of these two systems, has long been common (Bhatia et al. 1975). The degree of overlap will differ from culture to culture, possibly influenced by social complexity and the specialization entailed in it, much as described above in relation to the development of internalizing systems.

The distribution of the five types of skills across the sectors of health care and the degree of status attributed to them also will differ from culture to culture. However, skills that involve longer periods of training and the use of controlled substances or materials, or expensive, specialized technological devices with limited availability, are most likely to be confined to practitioners in Kleinman's (1986a [1978]) professional sector. Those skills involving everyday knowledge and locally available resources are likely to be used in the household production of health, Kleinman's popular sector (1986a [1978]). Where technology is idealized, those practitioners with technological skills may be vested with more authority than those who work with low-tech or no devices.

Herbalists treat people with or prescribe curative and preventive medicines made from plants. While many of the plants used can be classed as herbs, other plants, roots, bark, and other substances also may be made use of. Various plant parts can be prepared as teas or infusions to be drunk, or they can be kept in suspension in bottles of oil or alcohol, which will absorb various elements from them, and then can be used in small doses. Plants also might be ground down and mixed into pastes for external application. Some plants or plant combinations are smoked or absorbed through various body orifices, such as the nose.

A wide variety of foods are derived from plants, and so some practitioners classed as herbalists may make dietary recommendations. For example, the Jamaican condition called nerves, which comes about when a person's vital supply of sinews, a type of white blood, is depleted, can be treated with food supplements, as noted earlier. A diet rich in okra and other slimy foods, as well as liquidous foods light in color, is recommended.

While herbalists generally focus on plants, occasionally they may make recommendations related to nonplant foods. Herbalists also occasionally use minerals or other elements in their medicines, including vitamin supplements or maybe aspirin (derived from willow bark), but generally they do not use manufactured or isolated chemical compounds. Plants themselves and the ways they are used, rather than the isolated chemical compounds in them, are thought to be what effects a cure (see Etkin 1990).

Medicines made from isolated chemical elements are the domain of the **chemist** (this term is used in the United Kingdom to denote pharmacists). Chemists may rely on products that can be purchased over-the-counter to make their medicines or treatment recommendations; they also can, in some cases, prescribe controlled substances, as through a pharmacy (but not in a U.S. pharmacy, where diagnosing and prescribing are prohibited).

In certain economically poorer nations, we find chemists specializing in injections. Often the substance injected is a vitamin compound. The injectionist means to promote health, but unfortunately often s/he reuses unsterile needles, which is implicated in the spread of HIV infection and AIDS.

Another category of naturalistic practitioner is the **surgeon**, who cuts into the body to mend or alter it. Sometimes, s/he removes offending or diseased organs or substances from the body's inner reaches. Other times, the surgeon only cuts into the surface organs, as for blood letting or removing warts. While much surgery is corrective, other times it is preventive: male circumcision, for example, is thought by biomedical specialists to protect men against penile infection and women against cervical cancer. In certain regions of Africa, surgeons remove milk teeth as a preventive measure should a child be infected with tetanus or lockjaw; if this should happen, an oral portal will be open so that nutrition can be taken (Kate Hill, personal communication).

The **bodyworker,** or the musculo-skeletal specialist, manipulates the body to restore health. The category includes people who specialize in massage, bone setting, and skeletal realignment. The chiropractor, who is concerned with the latter, comes under this heading, as does the osteopath, who is also a biomedical practitioner, and the physical therapist. The Mexican *sobardor* is concerned with all the aspects of bodywork and may also massage the nerves and "cool the blood" to reduce swelling and inflammation, soften muscle and reduce pain and tension (Loustaunau 1990: 659).

The **midwife** works to bring about successful childbirth. The medicine midwives practice is primarily **preventive** and supportive and ensures, rather than restores, well-being. Generally, midwives are women who already have borne children of their own. Often, they learn their trade through a period of apprenticeship and may have specialized knowledge in all things related to reproduction, including abortion, contraception, and treatments for infertility. Sometimes, midwives take care of circumcisions as well.

In the United States, nurse midwives are distinguished from lay midwives. One category, both, or neither may be allowed to practice, depending upon state statutes. Much depends upon the local medical profession's perceived role of the midwife as related to biomedical practice (Eastman and Loustaunau 1987).

Special Blends

Practitioners of all five types work with the assumption that natural, pathophysiological bodily processes underlie the conditions they are treating. Sometimes, however, they may augment their naturalistic work with personalistic practices. So, in addition to the fact that both naturalistic and personalistic treatment practices can exist in one culture, one practitioner can draw on both types of technique. Some midwives, for example, may execute ritual actions to ensure that evil spirits do not trouble their pregnant charges or new mothers, as in the West Indian tradition. Sometimes this does happen, and midwives must drive the spirits away (or call in a personalistic specialist who can do so). In the United States, midwives often are seen as giving, in addition to naturalistic assistance, the personal and emotional support that is often absent in the biomedical approach to childbirth (Eastman and Loustaunau 1987).

The overt coexistence of both naturalistic and personalistic healing is evident in Jamaican tradition, where much medicine is naturalistic and sickness by default is seen as "natural." However, when a naturalistic treatment fails, when sickness after sickness befalls a person, or when a condition just does not seem typical or normal, personalistic etiology may be traced.

The coexistence of naturalistic and personalistic frameworks also is seen in the United States, with its officially naturalistic etiologies. Personalistic etiological notions are denigrated by the dominant culture, but nonetheless they are appealed to for answers that naturalistic etiological thought cannot provide: answers about the ultimate cause of sickness and suffering. As Irving Zola points out in relation to health surveys meant to determine how knowledgeable the public is about biomedical explanations,

We may be comforted by the scientific terminology if not the accuracy of [the respondent's] answers. Yet if we follow this questioning with the probe: "Why did you get X now?" or "Of all the people in your community, family etc. who were exposed to X, why did you get . . . ?", then the rational scientific veneer is pierced and the concern with personal and moral responsibility emerges quite strikingly. Indeed, the issue "why me?" becomes of great concern and is generally expressed in quite moral terms of what they did wrong. (1972: 491; ellipses in the original)

Similar findings are reflected in a study undertaken in Israel with mothers of children with Down's syndrome, which involves developmental retardation and is caused, according to biomedicine, by the existence of an extra chromosome. When the mothers explained the unusual birth outcomes, none mentioned chromosomes, despite the facts that education levels in Israel are generally high and biomedicine is the dominant medical system there. Instead, they talked of the stress of the Arab-Israeli war, family quarrels, bad dreams, and the like (Chigier, as cited in Moore et al. 1987 [1980]: 11).

Even where naturalistic etiologies or internalizing systems predominate, some sicknesses, perhaps especially new or ill-understood ones, such as AIDS, and ones associated with disfavored lifestyle choices, such as smoking or using narcotics, will be construed as punishments. Indeed, as Foster (1976) points out in regard to naturalistic and personalistic etiologies, the two are not mutually exclusive, and although a people may favor one over the other in general, both ways of understanding sickness will be present.

The degree to which these personalistic beliefs intrude on naturalistic systems varies considerably, from just a little (a U.S. surgeon saying that, in the end, the success of an operation is in God's hands; the midwife who wears an amulet to guard against evil) to a lot. When the threshold to "a lot" has been crossed, then that practitioner would probably be classed as subscribing to a personalistic model of treatment. The question to be asked in determining a classification is, "To which model is primacy given?" And to be able to gauge this, a better understanding of the personalistic mode is needed.

However, we should also note that because most traditions actually involve blends of both approaches, practitioners should try to meet clients' needs relating to both naturalistic and personalistic systems. One way to do this is by making sure to ask clients about concerns they may have regarding the downplayed dimension; for example, "What do you think is happening in your body?" or, in the case of the naturalistic practitioner, "Why do you think you caught it now?" A biomedical practitioner's ability to provide referrals, say to religious or spiritual specialists or to counselors, is important. No matter how well intended, an either-or position might be quite alienating. Even the staunchest supporter of biomedicine might need to feel s/he has an answer "why" when a loved one dies of a disease that generally does not kill or when someone who beat the odds of his or her condition last time succumbs this time around. It is extremely important for biomedical clinicians to have a basic understanding of personalistic systems and beliefs.

Personalistic Approaches

In contrast to naturalistic modalities, where sickness is an impersonal condition related to impersonal forces, **personalistic** approaches posit the intervention or influence of an active external agent. The agent may be human (e.g., a sorcerer) or nonhuman (e.g., an ancestral ghost, an evil force, or a deity). Accident or chance cannot account for sickness here as it can in a naturalistic explanation; sickness is the result of an agent's purposive act.

Sometimes, a person will find her- or himself the victim of a witch or other agent who purposefully chooses him or her as a victim through malice. But often, the purposive acts are provoked by the individuals who find themselves sick. That is, they are retributional acts. The agent involved in retribution might be a neighbor, angered by some antisocial behavior, an ancestral ghost put out by a lack of attention to his or her memory, or a punishing god, angered by a moral infraction. This is how sin can lead to sickness (Sobo 1993).

In personalistic systems, writes Foster, emphasis is placed on "the need to make sure that one's social networks, with fellow human beings, with ancestors, and with deities, are maintained in good working order" (1976: 780). For, if not retribution, behavior that is out of order surely will provoke at least a warning, in the form of ill health, meant to push one back into line. People fear this and so try to behave; the fear of sickness, or anxiety over the possibility of punishment for breaking social and moral rules, serves as a mechanism for maintaining social order (Hallowell 1977 [1941]: 132).

David Landy suggests that this fear "assumes the greatest generalized importance in those social systems in which there are few or no institutionalized and formalized mechanisms for settling disputes and enforcing conformity" (1977: 132). In other words, illness anxiety is most likely to serve a positive social function in simple, small-scale societies—societies in which, as Lewis (1986) and Young (1986 [1976]) note, no specialization or segregation of cultural domains, such that health systems function independently, has occurred.

Personalistic therapies hinge on the determination of why sickness happens; diagnosis, which Foster (1976) explains is more important than treatment per se, involves asking "Why?" or "Who is responsible?." Once an agent is identified, treatment steps can be taken. These steps vary widely across sociocultural contexts, individual case situations, and often even between healers in the same context depending on the background and healing preferences of each. Despite variation, because ideas about the social and moral order are entailed, personalistic healing generally involves religious action. It may also or otherwise involve the practice of magic.

Healing, Magic, and Religion

Magic, as defined in Whiteford and Friedl (1992: 316), "is the attempt to manipulate the forces of nature to obtain certain results." Magic effects a supernatural pressure on nature so that things that wouldn't normally happen do. The action (e.g., burning garbage gathered from one's home and chanting a spell to reverse cancerous growth) leads directly to the result.

Religion, on the other hand, generally holds that there are forces more powerful than humans in the universe and that these higher powers—not humans—control certain outcomes, such as whether a cure will be effective on certain kinds of illnesses. So in religious healing we must persuade god(s), spirits, or spiritual forces to grant a certain result or instigate a particular chain of events on our behalf. Our action (e.g., doing good deeds and praying for Jesus to reverse cancerous growth) leads the higher powers to consider bringing about the result. Magic does; religion asks.

Religious action, by definition, entails the adoption of a moral stance that is pleasing to the higher power(s) and may involve magical rites (e.g., the Jewish practice of marking the doorpost with a mezuhzah, or protective amulet; the Christian practice of reading the Bible aloud to rebuke evil spirits). When carried out in tandem with religious actions, magic is linked with ideas about a moral universe; however, it can be carried out in non-religious contexts.

The principles behind **magical healing** (and **sorcery**, as magic is called when used for vengeance or malicious ends, as in causing sickness) are relatively straightforward and were first described by James Frazer in 1922 (1942). He called them, respectively, the law of similarity and the law of contact. Both are linked to the human capacity for symbolic thought.

The law of similarity applies, for example, when sticking pins into a doll made to resemble an individual produces pain in that individual. It dictates that red medicine can be good for the blood or that leaves with spots might cure a rash. It can be applied by naturalistic healers as well as personalistic healers, and indeed it is. But the former sees this as consistent with the laws of nature, not as bending or manipulating them, so although they may apply the law of similarity, they do not do so in a magical fashion.

The second principle of magic, the law of contact (once in contact, always in contact), generally guides people's choice of healing materials, as when a Jamaican healer known to Sobo treated the worn nightgown of a hospitalized woman with certain concoctions in order to make the woman herself well. It explains how the blood of Jesus can cure or how a relic (a preserved piece of a saint's body) can have healing power. And it also explains why individuals from many cultures guard their body excretions or hair and nail clippings: evil magic (sorcery) for retribution can be worked using these substances.

Religion, on the other hand, generally does not support vengeance against community members or kin (although that outcome still might happen). Treatment advised will benefit all by restoring social harmony while healing sick individuals. Because religious healing is concerned with issues of morality, many religions leave vengeance to the gods or other powerful forces. This is not to say that religious people never seek revenge or consult sorcerers—they do—but religious teachings may discourage intra-community hate and destructive confrontations while encouraging reconciliation.

Just as there are two types of practitioners who heal using magic (magical healers and sorcerers), there are two types of religious healing specialists: the priest and the shaman. The **priest** undergoes formal training, and the power held resides in the office rather than the individual. The **shaman**, on the other hand, is powerful as an individual, and his or her power comes directly from the gods, spirits, or spiritual forces (Whiteford and Friedl 1992: 327). The priest can bring humans' messages or requests for healing to the higher power(s), while the shaman often brings the higher power(s) directly to the people, acting as a medium through which the power speaks, or as a diviner (328), revealing past actions connected with the illness event.

A priest praying with a hospitalized individual before an operation is helping him or her to ask for protection so that the surgeons, who are dealing only with the proximate cause of the illness and not the ultimate cause, which may be seen by the patient as having to do with sin or redemption, will get it right. Shamans, whose work is more dynamic, heal as instruments of the higher power(s). A faith healer who brings eyesight to the blind through the laying on of hands and chanting only does so because, in touching the blind individual, s/he serves as a conduit for a god's or a spirit's or spiritual force's healing power. Faith healers are, then, simply one type of shaman.

The Placebo Effect

Personalistic healing can effect organic cures without affecting the proximate cause of an illness directly. This happens through the **placebo effect**. This effect is well utilized in many complementary therapeutics and is not unknown in biomedicine, where cures or improvements are effected with inert substances given to a patient who believes them to be medication. For example, as much as 50 percent of analgesic pain relief is due to a placebo response (Watkins 1996: 56).

Norman Cousins (1981: 56) explains that in the United States the placebo takes the form of a prescription for medication and is necessary because we live in a culture that focuses on drug therapy; every patient has been socialized to expect a medicine for every symptom, even if the physician deems it unnecessary; the prescription is a major part of the healing ritual.

While placebos per se were often an overt part of medical practice in the past, physicians today are generally reluctant to use or even to discuss the use of the placebo; it is viewed as unethical and implies deceiving the patient (Shorter 1985: 245–46). However, the inert sugar pills of yesterday, claims Shorter, have been replaced by powerful drugs used for the same purpose—particularly tranquilizers and antidepressants—to cure by suggestion. When patients take prescribed medications not medically indicated, the placebo effect may still operate, but there will also be organic reactions since the substances ingested are not inert.

Edward Shorter (1985) relates numerous cases of patients demanding pills and prescriptions, which generally are filled. If one doctor refuses, the patient will just keep searching for another who will comply with his wishes. " 'Good medicine,' " says Shorter, "bends in the wind of patient expectations" (235).

Although there is much uncertainty as to exactly how the placebo effect works, the process is culturally relative, and its success relies on the patient's socialization, beliefs, and trust in the healer. Berton Rouéche, a medical reporter, finds that the placebo receives its power from the "infinite capacity of the human mind for self-deception" (quoted in Cousins 1981). As Jamaicans say, belief can cure, and belief can kill.

The pressure that cultural attitudes and understandings can exert on health cannot be underestimated—as many successful healers know. Therapeutically, the patient must have a role in anything that has to do with their health, illness, living, or dying (Zola 1983). A patient's trust in his or her physician may serve as a placebo-like therapeutic mechanism (Shorter 1985); however, under some conditions, and when too much trust is given at the cost of limiting the patient's willingness or ability to accept the responsibility for making choices, it may do more harm than good. The "manipulation of the patient" (238) and abuse of trust, even if thought to be in the patient's best interest, raises important ethical questions.

It is now recognized that placebos are not only psychotherapeutic props to be used when the patient demands medication that the physician believes unnecessary or even risky, but they can have actual physiological effects, altering body chemistry without side effects (Watkins 1996). Watkins points out, "they may directly activate brain-immune pathways without involving expectancy or subjective feelings" (59). Psychoneuroimmunology, which investigates the ways that higher cognitive centers and limbic emotional centers may serve to regulate the immune system with a concomitant effect on health and illness, is amassing evidence for direct physiological outcomes. The therapeutic power of placebos appears to be established—exactly how they work as well as the ethics of appropriate usage in biomedicine is not.

Emic and Etic Points of View

In classifying personalistic and naturalistic healing approaches, we can refer to the **emic**, or insider's point of view, as contrasted with the **etic**, or scientific outsider's supposedly objective, universalized way of seeing the world. While from an emic perspective, personalistic illness is being treated, naturalistic illness may also be inadvertently addressed. The organic contents of a personalistic medicine can and often do contain compounds that can knock out bacteria or otherwise help in healing. The important point is that the cure is not *seen* as hinging on naturalistic action, but, rather, on the actions taken to loosen the hold of illness as personalistically acquired. And when this is the case, we must classify the approach as personalistic.

The same rule can be applied in classifying some medicines that are thought to effect organic cures, but that outsiders might say work through personalistic action (e.g., through pleasing god or removing spirits from the body, or by the placebo effect). If practitioners and clients attribute the effectiveness of the treatment to naturalistic factors, then naturalistic medicine it is. As outsiders are always positioned in some sociocultural context and so are prone to judge health systems by their own criteria, the best approach is to take the emic point of view as the classificatory key for attaining the best possible understanding of the position of individual clients and of what they might be thinking—and doing—about their treatment regimens.

CONTEMPORARY U.S. MEDICINE: THE OUTER FRINGES

Systems of health care, as we have seen, are constantly in flux; they may borrow from others and change with opportunity and necessity. Even in biomedicine, new systems have emerged, for example, in borrowing from the vitalist branch of the equilibrium tradition. Vitalism involves a kind of energy or healing force which is activated to reestablish balance and harmony. Similar thinking is an essential part of most alternative or complementary healing practices (Kaptchuk 1996).

Once considered quackery by physicians and nurses, therapeutic touch (or hand-mediated energetic healing) is one therapy from a vitalist tradition that has strongly attracted members of the nursing profession. This is perhaps because nurses must typically deal with the whole patient in all degrees of suffering, and thus are more willing to look for anything that might relieve that suffering.

Therapeutic touch is based on a belief in a universal healing energy, which is activated through touch, use of the hands, and the focus of the mind. In Western science, the most closely related concepts are physicists' descriptions of quantum and electromagnetic fields, which closely resemble the descriptions of the vitalist systems. Although the therapy looks odd to our culturally conditioned eyes, sometimes involving waving the hands over another person, the results of application have been statistically significant (Slater 1996: 133). Although much research is needed on outcomes, the technique has produced demonstrable relief for real suffering in patients receiving chemotherapy and those suffering with asthma, migraines, and symptoms associated with HIV (133).

Suffering and Quackery's Appeal

Norman Cousins, in a film presentation based on his book *Anatomy of an Illness* (1979), describes a man suffering from terminal cancer and his wife, who had heard that vitamin C might improve his quality of life. When they questioned their family doctor on the subject, the doctor replied "quack, quack." Cousins berates the doctor for insensitivity and cruelty; moreover, he criticizes the doctor for so easily dismissing something that, even if it were not naturalistically efficacious, might have provided the couple with some feeling of control and comfort and would have done no harm.

The "quack, quack" response has been rather typical of physicians confronted with almost any form of therapy not sanctioned by the biomedical profession or considered "scientifically validated." But complementary modalities are widely used and can no longer be so easily dismissed. What, then, is quackery? Wardwell (1972) identifies **quacks** as members of a sub-group of the quasi-practitioners who "pretend" to be scientific but are not (264). Quackery's benefits are ascribed to natural, as opposed to super-natural, forces—claims meant to lend appeal as well as to deceive.

Of course, clients of biomedical practitioners may actually be deceived as to the scientific benefits of therapies they receive. Even the physician may be "deceived" in using a therapy that scientific investigation enthusiastically supports but later debunks as inefficacious. The overuse of antibiotics, un-necessary surgery, such as hysterectomies, Caesarean sections, and even heart bypass operations, are cases in point. This, however, is not quackery (nor is it really deceit). The best definition of quackery thus hinges on the *intent* to deceive.

Even so, there may be psychotherapeutic benefits from "quack" thera-pies. "Faith," states Wardwell, "can be as central to the healing power of an unscientific technique [or for that matter a scientific technique!] as to the healing power of God" (1972: 265). The benefits of a therapy, if they occur, reinforce the belief in and support of the therapy.

But when therapy involves profiteering and diverting clients from proven treatment, tragedy may result. In quackery, the client is cheated of financial resources, and potentially beneficial therapy is postponed or denied; quack treatment itself also may prove dangerous or harmful.

Despite its appeal, the idea that quackery grows out of and feeds on ignorance is not altogether true. People of all ages, cultures, socioeconomic status, and educational level can be victims. Those who are highly educated, in fact, seem just as prone to appeals of pain relief and cure, sexual potency, rejuvenation, unlimited energy, and a slim silhouette. People who are des-perately sick and for whom biomedicine has no answers, such as people with HIV/AIDS or incurable cancer, may feel that they have nothing to lose in searching out other alternatives. These people form a lucrative clientele for those who purposely exploit hope, misery, and desperation. After years of educational campaigns against quackery and impossible claims, the in-dustry is booming with products promising cures for everything from ar-thritis, cancer, and heart disease to diabetes, hypertension, and AIDS.

There is a fine line between protection from the dangers of quackery and the open-minded consideration of possible efficacy and the enlistment of complementary therapies in treating the whole person. Socioeconomic con-ditions within our society are creating pressure for a reevaluation of com-plementary modalities as both cost effective and efficacious when combined with biomedicine. But the label of "quackery" too broadly applied builds a wall between scientific biomedicine and any complementary therapies whose efficacy might be investigated and understood as offering additional help in addressing all of our needs related to health and illness, including psychological, emotional, spiritual, social, and physical ones.

Perhaps education, and even legislation, have failed to curtail quackery because they do not touch the root of the problem. People are not only multicultural, they are multidimensional; as long as biomedicine ministers to only one of those dimensions, people will search for additional or alternative means for fulfilling human needs. A truly complementary approach, one that blends biomedical and alternative modalities, would minister to all the aspects of human suffering and perhaps quackery would then lose much of its appeal.

Albert Schweitzer, after years of medical experience in Africa, observed that "The [indigenous healer] succeeds for the same reason all the rest of us succeed. Each patient carries his own doctor inside him. They come to us not knowing that truth. We are at our best when we give the doctor who resides within each patient a chance to go to work" (quoted in Cousins 1981: 69).

We may all carry that "doctor inside," but when really ill, we also must often seek help from those with further knowledge and expertise to help. In the next chapter, we will explore the currently dominant medical system and how cultural elements were vital in its development. We will also examine how biomedicine is very much a part of culture, as well as a culture in itself.

FOR DISCUSSION

1. How might the social structure of health care practice be described? Why might it (or why might it not) be a good idea to think of health care workers as occupying different social positions or sectors? What might these sectors be?

2. In what way does Galenic medicine survive in the current construction of biomedicine? List some examples of humoral-style views and practices that you have observed in biomedical settings. How are these different from humoral-style ideas and practices carried out in your home in the name of good health?

3. All health practitioners should fit into the two main groups and the nine subgroups offered in this chapter (five subgroups are naturalistic; four are personalistic). What criteria would you use to categorize a practitioner as belonging to one or the other main group? What criteria would you use to categorize her/him within that grouping? Make a list of practitioners that you have patronized and try to class them accordingly. What function does classification serve?

4. What are some of the reasons that people visit differing types of practitioners? What factors make them turn away from others? Discuss quackery and how, as a label, it affects the use and acceptance of various therapies.

5

Biomedicine: History, Culture, and Change

A series of events culminating in the Flexner report of 1910 resulted in establishing allopathic [biomedical] professional knowledge as the dominant form—a transformation that quickly deligitimized all other kinds of knowledge, putting the newly defined medical profession in a position of cultural authority, economic power, and political influence.... *The power of authoritative knowledge is not that it is correct but that it counts.*

[Brigitte Jordan 1993: 153–54; emphasis in original]

Goal: To examine the development of the American medical system, including its multicultural roots and related contributions, from an ethnohistorical perspective.

Goal: To understand the difference between the scientific paradigm and medical care per se and how they are both influenced by and a part of culture; to identify various cultural issues related to biomedicine, including its limitations, and to become familiar with related evolving arguments and models.

Science is generally taken for granted in the United States as the ultimate authority regarding what is true and what is not (Barnes 1985). The scientific paradigm is based upon the **scientific method** of investigation, which consists of observing, hypothesizing, and testing expected relationships and predicting outcomes, then revising expectations when discrepancies arise. The dominant system of medicine in the United States, biomedicine, is based upon this scientific paradigm.

But the **scientific paradigm** (a set of guiding assumptions, theories, and methods) is only one means of understanding the world and might also be considered ethnocentric. Allan Johnson (1996) offers the example of a Zen Buddhist, who considers all aspects of the observable and unobservable world as an integrated whole and rejects the idea that such a method of breaking things down into parts and studying their relationships can help to control or understand the world (3).

Still, science, as practiced through the scientific method, has allowed us to make great discoveries and to gain insights into and understanding of countless phenomena and has resulted in innumerable products and technologies that would have been impossible without it. It is precisely this argument that supports, and in fact requires, the teaching and application of the scientific method in the educational system.

However, limitations of the dominant scientific paradigm for medical care have become increasingly apparent. Like all cultural systems, the medical system is a human invention, linked to all other aspects of society. Science is only one element in medicine's shifting and evolving development and character. This chapter explores that development and character.

THE MULTICULTURAL BACKGROUND

The United States was settled by a great diversity of peoples. New arrivals faced the common problems of illness and disease, but brought with them their own perceptions and approaches to health, illness, and treatment. The modern American medical system thus derived from this multiculturally based diversity of folk traditions and practices and evolved into a dominative system based on the biomedical model (grounded in the scientific method). Hans Baer (1989) observes that this model duplicates American class, racial/ethnic, and gender relations and constitutes the standard by which all other medical systems are measured (1110).

The alternative folk-based or sectarian systems that did not fit this model were eventually excluded from the system. Only those philosophies and therapies validated by the scientific method and sanctioned by mainstream or orthodox medicine would be seen to have value in healing. American medical pluralism, however, persists in the diversity of alternative health care systems. Whether these systems remain on the fringe, disappear, become co-opted by the dominant system, or become integrated into a more inclusive system remains to be seen.

HISTORY, CULTURE, AND THE HEALTH CARE SYSTEM

History shows that numerous factors and events, evolving within a multicultural framework around a core of institutionalized patterns of values and beliefs, have influenced the direction and construction of the American health care system. Prior to the late nineteenth and early twentieth centuries, however, medical histories were not critical histories, but were written from a medical point of view and were read basically by doctors for information on how to treat patients (Sigerist 1960 [1947]). By 1929, when medicine was becoming more "scientific," the histories began to focus on the concerns of medical humanists, of how to maintain patient-centered traditions of the past in the face of scientific objectivism—concerns that still are with us today.

Within the last few decades, the questions addressed by medical historiography have begun to concern the role and nature of medicine within culture. Medical knowledge has come to include social history, involving relations with patients, moral systems, patterns of disease, meaning of illness, and social responses to disease. In addition, "The study of epidemic disease entailed an inquiry into how episodic and extraordinary medical events reflected and produced changes in the organization of cultural norms and values, institutions and intellect" (Brandt 1991: 202).

But medical history has often been constructed around the impressive and progressive accomplishments of science as a history of triumph over ignorance and suffering. Without question, the astounding progress of biomedical science has made life longer and better for most of us. However, the emerging ethnohistorical framework, with emphasis on social factors, gives us another view—one that helps to explain this progress at a more human level and to understand the myriad of problems that have accompanied it.

It has been widely shown that social forces shape or construct our perceptions of health, illness, and healing, a process known as social constructionism (Lupton 1994). There are numerous meanings and definitions of social constructionism within sociology and anthropology; however, we support the notion of a contextual construction, which recognizes biological realities, but stresses the social context. This approach considers the influences of both human interaction and political-economic factors on development and meaning of health, illness, and care, which also must include the traditional roots of the system (for an extended discussion of social constructionism and this approach, see Brown 1995).

ROOTS OF THE U.S. HEALTH CARE SYSTEM

Despite the existence of more sophisticated typological schemes, such as the naturalistic-personalistic typology introduced in chapter 4, the term "folk medicine" is generally used to designate health-related beliefs and practices of traditional societies. Folk medicine therefore might be defined by its contrast to modern, scientific medicine—the official medicine of the industrialized world. It is from folk, or "unofficial" medicine, however, that many patients derive their attitudes, values, and decisions about medical care in general (Hufford 1992: 14). The United States has been a multi-

cultural nation from the beginning, and "all medical traditions in the pluralistic cultural environment of the United States affect one another deeply
and constantly" (Hufford 1994: 117).

The stereotype of folk medicine as isolated from the mainstream is
therefore not at all correct. Folk and official medicine even share certain
metaphors. Both may view certain diseases as malevolent invaders that "attack" the body, which then mounts a defense to "fight off" or "drive out"
the invaders (Magner 1992: 12). Folk traditions represent "a universal set
of efforts to cope with illness in ways that go beyond—but do not necessarily conflict with—what modern medicine has to offer" (Hufford 1992:
15).

Another example of the similarities of folk and contemporary healing is
in the use of symbols. Symbolic healing was and is a part of folk practice
and can be seen as operant in all healing through a type of "universal" or
deeper structure at the psychological level, which utilizes "culturally specific
symbol imagery" (Dow 1986). Religious healing, magical healing, and
Western psychotherapy all incorporate versions of this common structure,
regardless of culture. Dow explains that "Symbolic healing becomes possible when a particularized mythic world exists [or is established] for both
the therapist [healer] and the patient and when the patient accepts the
power of the therapist to define the patient's relation to that world. The
therapist [shaman, healer, psychotherapist] then attaches the patient's emotions to transactional symbols and manipulates these symbols [to effect
healing]" (Dow 1986: 66).

Overlap of folk with biomedicine may also occur through diffusion or
appropriation. Medical **syncretism** is the process of one group's borrowing
or adapting medical remedies, knowledge, and techniques of treatment and
diagnosis of illness from another group (Laguerre 1987). Syncretism occurred, for example, when access to various European healing methods and
remedies familiar to colonists in the New World were limited or nonexis-
tent, and new diseases were encountered. Indigenous knowledge and therapies then became extremely important.

Native Americans, generally quite healthy before new diseases were introduced by Europeans (Kunitz 1983), had wide knowledge of the ailments
and remedies indigenous to their own environments. As historian Vogel
states, "Circumstances compelled the adoption of Indian medicine on the
frontier, but its influence did not stop there, or even at the seacoast; nor
did it end with the passing of the frontier" (1990: 5).

Twaddle and Hessler (1987) note that "The Native American healer frequently assumed the superordinate role of teacher and doctor to whites, an
almost quixotic notion according to modern conceptions that define Native
American healing as primitive and folksy" (177). Others took the view of
one highly biased medical historian, U.S. Army Colonel P. M. Ashburn,
that "the savage Indians and the Negroes contributed little or nothing of

value to any branch of medicine, and from them we received a mass of superstition and ignorance that reinforced and strengthened what we had brought from Europe, a heritage that still plagues us" (quoted in Vogel 1990: 6).

Although general Native American healing philosophies differ from white Western biomedical views of health and illness, and there is considerable variation across indigenous groups. Native American acquaintance with the physiological effects of a large number of drugs was extensive and formed the groundwork for the development of such modern medications as anesthetics, insulin, antibiotics, and even birth control pills (Vogel 1990). That knowledge—as well as techniques such as sweat baths, surgery, poultices, and mineral soaks—form an important legacy for American biomedical practice. Divergent philosophies and a Western ethnocentric orientation have blinded us to this heritage, causing us to lose "some of the ability to assess where we have been and where our medical care system is taking us" (Twaddle and Hessler 1987: 177).

When we do acknowledge the past, we typically do so with generic examples relating to Native American, European, African American, Asian, and Hispanic folk medicine. But these ethnic designations each refer to a wide variety of cultures, each with its own approach to health, illness, and medical care. Syncretism occurred among them, as well as between them and other populations with whom they had cultural contact. There was also an on-going adaptation to new geographical environments and resources for all immigrant cultures, as well as a complex and intricate relationship with social institutions, culture, and social structure.

Folk Contributions

There were many reasons for the preservation, adaptation, and use of diverse folk remedies in America during colonial times. First, very few physicians formally trained in European medical schools were available in the seventeenth-century American colonies. In addition, the philosophical foundations of colonial society were rooted in democratic and egalitarian ideals. The prevalent democratic, antielitist attitudes of the times supported the notion that the practice of medicine was a matter of common sense, to which all had access. Health care was generally provided within social networks and came out of oral traditions passed down through families and friends and was not seen as the property of an elite few who charged for their services. The family was the source of care, and women the main caregivers.

Rural isolation also necessitated self-sufficiency; households generally provided for all their own needs, including food, shelter, clothing, and health care. In any case, many people simply could not afford medical care from a physician. Since many people lived in isolated rural areas, they not only had to pay the doctor's fee, but also had to pay transportation costs that often amounted to more than the fee itself. In addition, considering the level of professional medical knowledge, doctors could generally offer little that people could not provide for themselves.

Another reason for turning to folk-based care was that, up until the late 1800s and the advent of a more scientifically based and predictibly beneficial medicine, seeking professional medical care involved a highly calculated risk, since almost anyone could become a doctor. A medical degree could be purchased quite cheaply.

Even though several states eventually passed perfunctory licensing laws, "in 1846 almost any man with an elementary education could take a course of lectures for one or two winters, pass an examination and thereby automatically achieve the right to practice medicine by state law" (Shryock 1966: [1947] 152). So, due to patient experience and doctors' reputations, few people had much faith in physicians' abilities. Even officially trained physicians could not always agree as to the proper methods and courses of treatment (as is still often the case today).

Folk medicine and self-care were most practical and quite simply necessary. When people did require additional care, however, there was a variety of theories, treatments, and practitioners from which they could choose.

The Sectarians

Various philosophies and approaches to medical care originating both at home and abroad were popular during the nineteenth century. Some were labeled sects due to their exclusionary nature, dogmatic attitudes, and the intense loyalty of their followers. The sects each claimed to have discovered the true nature of disease and illness and the proper approach to cure and healing. They may have arisen partly as a response to what were considered "heroic cures" and therapies of orthodox physicians, which included such unpleasant and potentially dangerous practices as bleeding, purging, vomiting, sweating, blistering, and liberal use of such mineral compounds as calomel (mild mercurous chloride), later found to be highly toxic (Sullivan 1994).

Primary among these early sectarian groups were the Thomsonians, the eclectics who were basically botanic doctors, and homeopaths. Osteopathy, Christian Science, faith healing, and chiropractic appeared around the turn of the century and into the 1900s, as new sects replaced old (for an extended discussion of these medical sects, see Micozzi 1996b).

Abraham Flexner (1910), in his classic assessment of the status of American medical education (to be discussed later), saw sects as an inevitable and even logical opposition to preconceived notions (other than their own) about causes and treatments for illness. Orthodox medical philosophy and practice, termed allopathic medicine, was, at the time, just as sectarian as the rest (Starr 1982). Flexner felt that with the establishment of a scientific basis for diagnosis and treatment, all philosophies would be submitted to rigorous scientific examination. He predicted that the sectarian approaches would either die out (their schools in the United States were already reduced, and enrollment was declining) or be co-opted into the modern medical fold. His predictions were to prove only partially correct (Starr 1982).

The Orthodox Profession of Medicine

In colonial times, doctors (those trained in or possessing some official medical knowledge, who identified themselves as physicians), especially those trained in Europe, viewed the practice of medicine as a basis for social status and aristocratic privilege rather than a profession to serve those in need. The title "physician" thus entailed aristocratic patronage from the wealthy and powerful and legal protection as practitioners—benefits and privileges that were simply not available to doctors in a democratically inclined American colonial society where equality was the ideal.

Doctors in America therefore found themselves in competition with lay practitioners, folk medicine, and eventually other (sectarian) systems of therapy. Doctors also competed with **patent medicine** companies, which sold their trademarked medical preparations directly to the public, offering their own explanations of causes and easy cures for a multitude of ailments from arthritis to baldness.

Competition was augmented by the fact that the demand for physicians was essentially low at the same time that physicians, due to the lax restrictions on entry into the field of medicine, were in oversupply. By 1846, due to strong competition, "The excess of physicians was such that many young graduates failed to secure a decent practice and abandoned the profession" (Shryock 1966: 156).

Some doctors declared that medical discoveries should be disseminated to the lay public in easily understood language, thereby providing the lay public with greater self-healing knowledge. Other doctors, however, saw medicine as a privileged profession, with specialized knowledge that conferred status and should not be shared with those who could not understand its complexities. This position reflects an early attempt to use **authoritative knowledge**—knowledge that "builds and reflects power relationships"—to construct a stronger professional base and what Jordan calls a "community of practice" (1993: 153). Drawing on the work of various social theorists, Jordan relates this move to autonomy to a cross-culturally identified process,

whereby the authority of [a] particular knowledge system and the power relations supporting it and benefitting from it come to be perceived not as socially constructed, relative, and often coercive, but as natural, legitimate, and in the best interest of all parties. . . . This process makes the achieved order of the world appear to be a fact of nature, with the consequence that the dominant positions in that order are also a fact of nature, and hence cannot be changed [Jordan 1993: 153].

While physicians established a position of status and privilege through professional identity and licensure, science was to provide a more solid foundation and open the way to a "legitimate" complexity, moving professional medicine out of the realm of lay understanding and common sense and, ultimately, to complete professional autonomy.

Science, however, was only one link in the chain of events. Paul Starr (1982) links the development of the modern medical system with the rise and increasing dominance of the medical profession in the United States, and notes that professional dominance was actually achieved before science had contributed much to the doctors' capabilities for addressing disease. Early scientific discoveries were important, but made little impact on actual medical care. Practicing physicians had little to offer their patients until the catalyst of World War II.

One physician, Dr. J. Dunbar Shields, recalled his frustration with the impotence of medicine before World War II. He could envision enormous possibilities, but described the time as "an era of very little light" and remarked upon the need to sit down with the patient and listen—"to comfort and console always" (quoted in Kaufman 1993: 151)—since in most cases, doctors could do little else. Another internist, Dr. Saul Jarcho, describing his practice between 1936 and 1942, observed, "For cases of infection, there were no antibiotics when I first started in practice. I would try to support the patient's nutrition and morale and physical cleanliness. . . . Almost all organic diseases of the nervous system were untreatable" (quoted in Kaufman 1993: 161). This emphasizes the importance of nonbiomedical factors in the achievement of dominance by the biomedical system.

GROWTH OF THE SCIENTIFIC MEDICAL MODEL

A number of significant discoveries and events are generally cited as instrumental in establishing the centrality and dominance of scientific medicine, which consequently discredited other systems of healing. Louis Pasteur's germ theory of disease, the founding of the American Medical Association, Abraham Flexner's Report on the State of American Medical Education, and the development of the hospital system, plus later rapid growth of technology after World War II, had major cultural impacts upon treatment modalities and the context and delivery of health care in the United States.

The Germ Theory

In the 1860s and 1870s, Louis Pasteur, a French chemist, isolated the organisms responsible for major infectious diseases, including deadly rabies. His formulation of the germ theory had a tremendous impact upon a broad range of scientific medical research and development (Magner 1992).

The **germ theory**, initially embraced as *the* primary explanation for the spread of disease, was powerful, appealing, and simplistic. Once accepted, the theory generated a great deal of enthusiasm and stimulated the search for disease-causing germs. But the idea that germs are monocausal agents (one germ for each disease) proved to be in error. For a time, the blind acceptance of this idea kept researchers from exploring other avenues of causation, such as additional pathological, social, cultural, and environmental factors that turned out to be vital to understanding and controlling the disease process. At this time, patients' cultural backgrounds, beliefs, values, and traditions were considered inconsequential to diagnosis and treatment.

The germ theory achieved great advances; it changed causal attribution and related practices and added to knowledge about the sources of contagion and the health-and-illness connections between and among communities and even nations. Diseases could now be scientifically classified according to perceived causes rather than only signs and symptoms, and illness was no longer explained only by physical or social conditions or as a divine punishment for moral infractions. After the germ theory, however, "The culture of the organism, not of the patient, was the important determinant of sickness" (Kunitz 1994: 176).

The American Medical Association

Even before the discovery of germs, physicians pursued their quest for control and professionalization of medicine. They established medical societies in some states during the first half of the nineteenth century, and in 1847, they met in Philadelphia to establish the American Medical Association (AMA). This was a key step in the professionalization process. A reorganization of the AMA in 1902 established branch societies on the local, state, and territorial levels. Local societies had the arbitrary discretion to expel or deny membership to any physician, and thus could determine membership qualifications and enforce conformity. This enabled the profession to monitor and control a widely dispersed membership.

Having a professional association allowed physicians to better organize their attack on competitive elements, as well as to further develop the scientific basis for medicine and the legitimacy of the scientific approach. They still disagreed with and battled each other on all sorts of medical, philosophical, and organizational issues, but the AMA provided a forum where interests could be discussed and defended, and also served as a potential pressure group for future political and policy endeavors.

Richard Shryock (1966) compared the status of the profession in the late 1940s to its status 100 years previously. From newspaper headlines and articles of the earlier times, it was evident that the early status of the medical profession was not at all high; the editor of the *Cincinnati Medical Observer* of 1857 was quoted as pointing out that many "speak of the Medical Profession as a body of jealous, quarrelsome men, whose chief delight is in the annoyance and ridicule of each other" (quoted in Shryock 1966: 151). It wasn't until near the turn of the century that the status of members of the American medical profession really began to improve. Its potential power by that time, however, was considerable.

The power of the AMA was used to raise and maintain academic and scientific standards, but it was also used to consolidate power and further its own interests, including the economic position of the medical profession. It also helped to secure the autonomous right to define and enforce the restraints, as well as the standards of practice, with a freedom known to very few professions. Thus, there emerged what Freidson called "a new tyranny which sincerely expresses itself in the language of humanitarianism and which imposes its own values on others for what it sees to be their own good" (1970: 382).

Another event supporting professional dominance occurred in 1910 with the publication of the Flexner Report. A broader view of that event reveals not only its role in the establishment of scientific medicine and standardized medical education, but its links with social-structural, capitalist cultural values as well.

The Flexner Report

In 1908, the AMA contracted with the Carnegie Foundation for a study of American medical education to be conducted by Abraham Flexner, an administrator and educator. The goal of the study was to standardize and raise the status of American medical education. Since the cost of a scientific medical education was beyond most students, and capital investment and operating costs for schools were beyond the means of the profession, it was recognized that the money would have to come from the rich. Both philanthropists and the public would therefore have to be convinced that modern medicine was a field worthy of their support.

Professional medical reformers were well aware of the need for a strategy consistent with current historical forces. This meant offering investment opportunities in conquering disease and the promise of international status and leadership to investors (E. Brown 1979: 141). In keeping with the new scientific discoveries and inventions in the industrial sector, which promised growth and profits, the time had come to promote "scientific medicine."

The resulting **Flexner Report** of 1910 is generally cited as an historical turning point in medical education (e.g., Chase 1973). The movement for medical school reform, however, had actually begun in 1870 at Harvard. The AMA's Council on Medical Education had even done a preliminary survey in 1907, which served as the basis for Flexner's report, and state medical boards had already begun to upgrade medical school programs (Brown 1979). The report did force the closure of numerous medical schools judged to be of inferior quality, although due to previous competition and the push for reform, as many schools had closed before as after the report was issued. Unfortunately, many of those schools closed had trained women and other minorities.

Before 1910, medical education was open to women in the United States and Canada practically on the same terms as to men. Any woman who desired a medical education should have no difficulty in finding a school, asserted Flexner (1910). With fewer schools and increased competition, however, a growing male hostility within the profession led to policies of women's exclusion. In the matter of medical education, now required for licensure and credentials, "Administrators justified outright discrimination against qualified women candidates on the grounds that they would not continue to practice after marriage" (Starr 1982: 124). Medical schools for the next half century after 1910 maintained quotas limiting women to about 5 percent of admissions (124).

A product of a racist society, Flexner supported the medical training of Blacks, but only in order to care for other Blacks—not because they themselves needed care, but because they also came into contact with Whites. He emphasized their educational need to concentrate on hygiene rather than surgery. He recommended that out of seven schools for Blacks, two schools, Meharry and Howard, be supported and upgraded and the others eliminated. The reduction in black schools resulted in decreased care for Blacks. In 1910, there was one black physician for every 2,883 black people in the United States; by 1942 the ratio was one black physician for every 3,377 black people (Brown 1979: 154).

The Flexner Report had positive consequences in educating the public to the benefits of scientific medicine and medical training by standardizing medical education and eliminating the medical diploma mills, which in turn reduced the risk of unproven, incompetent, or fraudulent treatment. However, the report also allowed the medical profession to more closely guard its gates against all but the elite few allowed to become physicians.

With the establishment of uniformity in medical training for all students, and with more uniformity in students themselves (the licensed, medical workforce consisted mostly of white, upper middle-class males), the profession became more homogeneous. Higher costs of a medical education, plus the extended time necessary for study and certification, limited the entry of lower and working classes. Places in medical schools became scarce and competition for them resulted in policies of discrimination against Jews, Blacks, women, and immigrants. Exclusion from the mainstream meant that alternative philosophies and ideas of diagnosis and treatment could be effectively controlled or suppressed or could be consigned to a lower class or ethnically identified population. The exclusionary race-class-sex composition of the profession persisted until the opening up of medical education with affirmative action programs in the 1960s and 1970s, and had profound consequences for the development of the health care system in the United States.

The Flexner Legacy

Taking into account the larger context and social dynamics of the time, the Flexner Report can be seen as an attempt by the AMA to "attain and maintain ideological hegemony over the other sects of medicine that were still extant at the time"; it also helped to "solidify the alliance between the capitalist class and the AMA and to establish the dominance of the re-searcher over the practitioner" (Berliner 1975: 589). Further, the report established a new medical paradigm—that of the body as machine with an emphasis on research, therapy, and repair (pathology and cure). "That this conception . . . is a reflection of the larger economic system is not to be considered an accident" (590).

Berliner's conclusion (as well as the similar conclusions of others, e.g., Martin 1987; Zola 1983; Baer 1989) is based on the presence of vested capitalist interests in legitimating the existing social structure of the times, with its emphasis on scientism, and the subordination of means of produc-tion, including medical care institutions, to capital accumulation. Imple-mentation of the Flexner Report was undertaken by the nine largest philanthropic organizations in the United States, which together gave over $150 million to particular medical schools over the twenty years following the emergence of the Report (Berliner 1975: 590). These organizations had strong ties to their industrialist sponsors and reflected their interests.

In the pre–World War II era, philanthropic foundations contributed to strengthening medical schools, biomedical research, and public health pro-grams. In 1940, foundation grants totaled $12 million, or 30 percent of the total national expenditures in this area. In the postwar era, however, philanthrophic donations were far outstripped by funding from private in-surance; federal, state, and local governments; and consumer out-of-pocket payments. Thus it can be argued that the foundations have not been the "movers and shakers" they were thought to be (Ginzberg 1990). Still, the early alliance of medicine with wealthy capitalist interests profoundly af-fected the development of the system. Large investments are not made with no thought to hope of return. Many within the AMA recognized the dan-gers of alliances with strong capitalist interests who would then have a say in designating areas of priorities in education and research (Brown 1979). These areas could be chosen to provide investment opportunities with bigger payoffs and to support the class structure rather than according to need. As Berliner suggests, "The problems that plague the field of medicine today no doubt emerge dialectically from the attempt made in 1910 to shore up a medical system also beset with contradictions and conflicts" (1975: 590).

The Development of the Hospital System

Hospitals also played a role in the growth and dominance of mainstream medicine. They provided a laboratory for the science of medicine and for the physician's practice, creating an institution that would become central to the medical care delivery system.

Before 1850, hospitals served the indigent poor and acute cases or short-stay patients, while chronic cases, the incurable, the insane, and those with communicable diseases were sent to public institutions through a form of rationing. These people were not considered appropriate subjects for hospital admissions, and would take up space that might be better used by those who could be cured or benefit from treatment (Rosen 1974).

In the mid–nineteenth century, various religious or ethnic institutions were developed for specific diseases such as tuberculosis, for categories of the population such as women and children, and for various medical sects such as homeopathy. These specialty hospitals served several purposes: they offered internships and residencies for minority physicians who were denied entry elsewhere, and they allowed them a facility for attending their patients. Specialty hospitals also eased the fears of various religious and ethnic minorities, that cultural customs, beliefs, and rituals—such as last rites, confession, or kosher diet requirements—would not be honored or would be ridiculed in traditional general hospitals.

Cultural separatism offered at least some opportunity for educational advancement and sensitive, culturally relative care for minority populations, but at a price: it did nothing to change the discriminatory structure of society and social institutions or to lessen the intolerance and insensitivity of health care providers toward other cultural groups. Separatism served a stabilizing function by not upsetting the socially dominant, very "unscientific" racist and ethnocentric structure (see Krause 1977).

The development of the American hospital system was basically unplanned, with no conscious efforts at coordination, but it did reflect a definite pattern of class relations (Starr 1982). This was especially true in the elite private hospitals where staff were strictly controlled and patients were either very poor (for teaching purposes) or very rich (for revenue). The centralization of both learning and practice within a hospital setting made it much easier to maintain a particular standard of medical education with control of curriculum, training, and requirements. The role of the hospital, however, changed and continues to change, linked to social and economic forces and historical events. A major change, for example, occurred with the advent of World War II.

WORLD WAR II: A TURNING POINT

By the 1940s, the power of the dominance of biomedicine was more or less secured. However, the war made scientific medicine a national asset and an institution, and served as a catalyst for a boom in scientific research that would further define the culture of scientific medicine. Research produced medical discoveries that lowered the military death rate and could be translated to the populace. The United States emerged from the war as a formidable economic and military power. Scientific medicine became associated with victory, the conquest of infectious diseases, prosperity, and leadership of the free world—biomedicine was American.

The 1940s and 1950s were what might be termed the golden age of antibiotics. The physicians' arsenal for combating disease was filled to overflowing with new miracle drugs, and the military metaphors used in descriptions of medical victories over disease fit nicely with the victory coming out of World War II. Penicillin, whose research and development was closely associated with military needs and objectives, proved to be effective against venereal diseases as well as battle injuries, and streptomycin was found to be effective against tuberculosis. These advances fueled the search for new drugs and their potential profits.

The new, scientifically tested and approved medications were dramatic and impressive, but diverted attention from and further discredited folk remedies and traditional forms of medical care. Use of the new drugs became a status symbol, while folk practices became associated with ignorance and superstition. Biomedicine developed a heavy reliance upon new drug therapies for treatment and cure, in spite of early warnings that overuse and misuse of antibiotics could produce dangerous side effects and drug-resistant strains of bacteria. These warnings have unfortunately proven to be correct (see Garrett 1994). The use of scientifically developed and approved drugs as a major medical therapy, however, was firmly established.

The field of psychiatry also emerged from the war with newfound status and began to define social problems and conditions in medical terms. Various areas that had previously not been considered as medically related, such as depression, began to be viewed as medical problems to be treated. This viewpoint was supported by an alliance of liberalism (which was focused on promoting the public good) and biomedicine (since it broadened the need for medical research, hospital construction, and other forms of resource development) (Starr 1982).

With postwar economic growth and prosperity, the advance of scientific medicine promised health and well-being through progress without any need for a restructuring of society. Government supported the programs, but specifically refrained from any intervention in policy. Since definition of the concept of a "profession" was considered to require autonomy (Turner 1995), this development was not inconsistent with prevailing cultural and political beliefs.

The public service orientation of biomedicine, its ethical basis, and claim of specialized knowledge actually justified nonintervention (no regulation) by government. The Marxist interpretation that professional groups (including medicine) under state protection actually support the capitalist enterprise by legitimizing conditions of production (including health) through monitoring and maintaining surveillance of the working class (Turner 1995: 130; also see Foucault 1975 [1963]) would also justify nonintervention by the state. The emerging structure of the United States' dominant medical system thus remained intact.

CRISIS AND REFORM

The Road to Alternatives

The belief in growth without conflict continued until the 1960s, when the flaws and cracks in the biomedical system began to grow apparent. The goal of biomedicine was challenged as people who recognized the benefits and need for medical care could not afford it. The system responded to needs in an ad hoc fashion, if at all.

The mainstream biomedical system that had evolved by the 1970s was still loosely aligned and basically uncoordinated. Never designed to serve the poor, it was profession-dominated, scientifically based, cure-oriented and hospital-centered, with an open, unregulated fee structure. It was also "overly specialized, overbuilt and overbedded, and insufficiently attentive to the needs of the poor in inner-city and rural areas" (Starr 1982). Health care facilities were unevenly distributed, with resulting inequity in services provided. Physicians tended to opt for practice in wealthier urban areas where large hospitals offered high-tech educational facilities and opportunities, interaction with colleagues, and higher incomes. This resulted in duplication of services in some areas, with few or no services in others.

A two-tier system of care had been created, clogging emergency rooms and placing a burden on public hospitals with the poor and indigent and raising issues of ethics and inequitable quality of care. Many rural and inner city areas had virtually no access to health care at all. A growing shortage of **primary care physicians** (those who see the patient first), which resulted from increasing medical specialization, also limited access to family doctors who knew their patients and could coordinate their care.

Three independent national surveys, supported by the Robert Wood

Johnson Foundation in 1976, 1982, and 1986, examined the extent of difficulties for individuals seeking medical care. It was found that from 1982 to 1986, even though health status for both Blacks and Hispanics was poorer than for Whites, these groups were significantly less likely to be hospitalized. In addition, "an estimated one million individuals actually tried to obtain care but did not receive it. The majority of Americans experiencing these difficulties were the poor, uninsured, or minorities" (Freeman et al. 1990: 316). The emerging value of health care as a "right" carried no accompanying responsibilities for providing it.

The Corporate Incursion and Consumer Activism

Perhaps the greatest challenge to biomedical professional dominance has come from within the very nature of the capitalist system itself. The history of the growth of corporate (for-profit) medicine, too long and complex to include here, raises the question of whether medicine with the primary emphasis on profit is or can be consistent with the service orientation of medicine as it relates to the good of humanity and the alleviation of suffering.

By the 1960s and 1970s, biomedicine had the potential of a growth industry, but with increasing costs and poor management, it was floundering. Corporate entry brought with it much needed capital investment and management techniques for securing a profit (Wohl 1984). The view of biomedicine as a profit-making enterprise, however, has further distanced it from a service orientation, and such a philosophy is in direct conflict with the goal of providing care for those who cannot pay. Doctors find themselves not only at odds with their own patients, but with the corporate entities who, unlike the government, demand a monetary return on their investments. Professional autonomy becomes co-opted and weakened as doctors find themselves captives of the corporate bottom line.

The 1980s and 1990s have seen attempts to restructure the system with health maintenance organizations, group practice, managed care, and other means to hold down costs. With access to medical care a growing concern, however, consumers have become disaffected with the biomedical profession and the still-rising cost of care. The expected service orientation clashes with the view of physicians as wealthy entrepreneurs, living off of the misery and desperation of the sick.

There has also been a resultant explosion of consumer knowledge with the wide availability of books, newsletters, television programs, and public classes, all for the purpose of educating the population with regard to prevention and care; many of these efforts have been sponsored by, written by, or feature physicians. The early advocacy of self-help has reappeared— not so much as common sense, but as personal interest in education and knowledge aimed at health maintenance and illness prevention and gaining more control in consumer decision-making (Salmon 1984: 220).

Consumers have also rediscovered and are showing great interest in what are considered **alternative** or **complementary** systems, or forms, of care. They may be used instead of, but are more generally used in conjunction with, mainstream therapies. Many of these additional systems of health care have simply coexisted with biomedicine like islands in the medical mainstream. Herbs, massage, chiropractic, acupuncture, homeopathy, faith healing, and other therapies offer alternatives when biomedical care is un-affordable, unobtainable, or unsatisfactory. Many of these alternatives have remained primarily within subcultural groupings of poor racial and ethnic minorities, but are by no means limited to them.

A study at the University of Pennsylvania Cancer Center found that 13 percent of cancer patients, mostly white and well-educated, were also using one or more folk medical treatments for their illness (Cassileth et al. 1984). A more recent study published in the *New England Journal of Medicine* found evidence that about one in every three Americans uses alternative treatments, but most don't tell their doctors (Eisenberg et al. 1993).

There is little argument that the American health care system is in need of reform. The United States is the only Western industrialized nation that does not have some form of **universal health care** (basic care for all or a large majority of the population). The challenge is not only to make the system cost effective and to provide for the health care needs of all the people to the greatest extent possible, but to make the system more tolerant of and responsive to other cultural values and approaches, which as we will see is vital in the production of health and prevention and treatment of illness.

This would mean moving away from the biomedical model as the single acceptable approach to a more integrated and inclusive model that considers the patient as a whole multidimensional person and affirms that healing is psychological, social, spiritual, and cultural, as well as biological. Such a shift would, in turn, entail some major structural changes in the face of not only biomedical but also corporate interests vested in the present system, as well as the real value structure and belief system of the U.S. population.

However, the upsurge in use of alternative medicines does not necessarily mean the beginning of a more medically pluralistic system: "As long as the corporate class and its state sponsors dictate health policy, the American medical system will remain a dominative one and continue to reflect social relations in the larger society" (Baer 1989: 1111). It is therefore necessary to understand biomedicine as a part of culture and as a culture in itself, as well as understanding its relationship to cultural needs and perceptions.

BIOMEDICINE IN CULTURE

Constructing Disease, Illness, and Medicine

Almost no one doubts that there is a biological reality. When the normal structure or functioning of the body is disrupted by a disease condition, such as a malignant tumor, it is certainly "there." It can be seen (as through imaging or surgery) and felt (as in symptoms and pain), and it can cause the death of the organism it inhabits or affects. A broken bone is broken; arteries can be plugged; and variations in blood pressure and body temperature can be measured.

Disease conditions can be medically interpreted and treated in numerous ways with some predictibility of outcome; some conditions can be cured, some controlled, and others alleviated or made bearable. To an individual, however, a broken bone or a tumor means far more than a simple pathology. A subjective person, not an objective organism, suffers. This is the crux of the failure of modern medicine.

Sociologist Ann Holohan describes her reaction to the threat of a possible malignant breast tumor and the doctor's announcement of the need for a biopsy:

I got up, struggled to preserve normality (this seemed enormously important) and was astonished to hear myself asking mundane questions about admission procedures for tomorrow. He opened the door and still in a state of utter turmoil, I walked into the street. It seemed incredible that nothing had changed—the sun was still shining, the road sweeper gathering the leaves. I sat in my car, and with the conventional constraints removed, immense waves of panic engulfed me. I drove blindly home and recall very little of the actual journey. I felt this alien, pathological change was inexorable, gone was the reassuring external cause of my symptoms. Yet clearly I was no "sicker" than before my consultation. All that had changed was the possibility of a medical label for my symptom. (1977: 87–88)

As it turned out, Holohan did not have cancer; the tumor was benign. But the possibility and the meaning of that possibility for her elicited psychological and physical reactions far beyond the lesion, which was not producing any alarming symptoms at the time.

Many cultural influences contributed to her reactions, including her perceptions of vulnerability, what she knew and did not know about cancer, the attitudes of friends and others toward the disease, her degree of trust in the doctor's diagnostic and treatment abilities, and her perception of the disruption of her life, including the threat to end it. In addition, she would have to consider the cost of unguaranteed survival—in financial terms, depending upon insurance coverage and personal resources, in personal time lost, pain and suffering, and the effects on her family. She would have to deal with the medical system—the possible treatment modalities, the options presented to her, and the vital importance of her doctor's and her own decisions based upon an estimation of odds.

In terms of meaning, then, we are dealing with two typologies, both of which may be socially and culturally constructed: the patient's expectations and experience of personal and social effects on her life (**illness**) and the physician's experience of treating a concrete biological entity (**disease**). To say that a disease is "socially constructed" does not necessarily deny the biological reality of the disease (Lock 1988). It does, however, recognize that the meaning of the illness for both healer and patient derives from its historical, cultural, and individual, as well as biological, context (Brandt 1991: 204).

It has generally been assumed that clinical diagnoses and decision-making on the part of physicians takes place in a clinically autonomous environment, is objectively based on signs and symptoms, and is isolated from the social milieu. In an extensive literature review of the role of social structure in clinical decision-making, however, Clark, Potter, and McKinlay (1991) noted the influence of preconceived ideas of providers that, for example, result in the underdetection of coronary heart disease in women. As an illustration, a 40-year-old patient presents with chest pain. Since women who have not yet reached menopause are considered to be at one-third the risk of heart disease as men, and since American women generally get their primary care from a gynecologist whose focus is not on the cardiovascular system, heart disease is much less likely to be suspected if that patient is female rather than male.

However, the Framingham study, one of the most extensive studies ever to be undertaken in relation to heart disease, using age-adjusted data, showed that women have nearly 50 percent more silent heart attacks, have higher case fatality rates, and present with more advanced or severe heart disease than men (Clark, Potter, and McKinlay 1991: 862). Thus, the researchers conclude that "Research designs should now go further in specifying the linkages between physicians' thinking, their interaction with patients, and the wider social structure" (862).

Involvement of social factors may also be discerned in P. Brown's "sociology of diagnosis" (1995), a typology of conditions and definitions that uses four basic designations. "Routine conditions," covering the vast majority, are easiest to diagnose, least conflictual, and involve primarily an adjustment and adaptation on the part of the patient, who may reject the diagnosis due to its disruptive potential. "Medicalized definitions" involve conditions that are generally nonmedical where biomedical definitions are applied. Medical labeling here may be a form of social control or professional expansion or may be a source of legitimation for many vague conditions such as chronic fatigue or pain syndromes. "Contested definitions" are those that may be widely accepted, but with no accompanying applied clinical medical definition, such as in the case of chemical contamination of military personnel during the Persian Gulf War. This hesitancy for medical confirmation may arise out of rigid diagnostic criteria, opposition to lay involvement in diagnoses, and fear of political and economic consequences. Finally, "potentially medicalized definitions" are those conditions not currently medicalized, but that may be so in the future, such as genetic predispositions, identified through screening. These conditions are not in themselves medical conditions, and they may never become such (P. Brown 1995: 40–42). Nevertheless, "These screening approaches wind up defining as pathology the genetic makeup, rather than the disease that may arise" (42). Possible consequences are workplace exclusion policies, where the victim is blamed for a predisposition, and exclusion from insurance coverage.

Biomedicine and the Dominant Capitalist Culture

Biomedicine evolved out of a tradition of service to suffering humanity, an ideal value strongly supported in the United States. The developing structure of the American biomedical system, however, supported and was consistent with the values of capitalist enterprise, as we have seen. Common elements included the struggle for status and control, competition for markets, and political maneuvering of vested capitalist interests. The basic environment was one of marketplace medicine, where clinical services were sold to the patient for a fee by a practitioner in private practice.

The capitalist connection was even more apparent when biomedicine, in the 1960s, responded with fierce resistence to the implementation of the government-sponsored programs of Medicare and Medicaid, which provide funds for care for the aged and the poor, respectively. Milford O. Rouse, a former president of the AMA, was quoted by Ashley Montagu in a letter to the *New York Times* in 1969: "We are faced with the concept of health care as a right rather than a privilege. . . . What is our philosophy? It is the faith in private enterprise. We can, therefore, concentrate our attention on the single obligation to protect the American way of life. That way can be described in one word: Capitalism" (Montagu 1969).

The seeming contradiction of service versus profit is one of the perennial dilemmas of the medical profession; if the free enterprise system is incapable of providing care for all those who require it and care is to be conceived of as a right rather than a privilege, then how, and by whom, is it to be delivered and financed? The 1960s introduction of the Medicare and Medicaid programs was a recognition that rising costs and restricted access required government intervention.

Although the AMA denounced both Medicare and Medicaid as threats to private enterprise and "the American way," Medicare was ultimately rationalized as acceptable through the input of social security payments and inclusion of payment of physicians' fees. Medicaid, however, since it was directed to the poor and was left to the states to determine the extent of programs, was underfunded and, therefore, much less lucrative. It was also seen as a less legitimate form of public assistance in a capitalist society, and physician participation was far more limited (Starr 1982).

In the 1960s, the growing emphasis on health care as a right, as well as the perspective that illness could be and was socially engendered, involved conceptual shifts, but did not demand structural ones. Renee Fox (1977) wrote that discussions regarding the destratification of the physician's role and the concept of national health insurance in the 1970s actually reaffirmed the traditional American values of equality, independence, self-reliance, universalism, distributive justice, solidarity, reciprocity, and individual and community responsibility (21).

Still, Fox predicted little change in the overall structure of health care, noting that in spite of trends toward increased appreciation of personal and communal health, the influences on health of personal behavior, greater use of nonphysician professionals, and greater emphasis on prevention, "none of these trends implies that what we have called cultural demedicalization will take place." By this, Fox meant that health, illness, and medicine would remain central preoccupations of the society, and that they would maintain the "social, ethical, and existential significance they have acquired" (21). Thus far, this seems to be the case. Biomedicine as a part of culture essentially incorporates, supports, and reflects both the ideals and realities of society in its philosophies and functions. Even science itself, the foundation on which the dominant medical institution and the practice of biomedicine rests, reflects social realities and is open to cultural interpretation.

How "Scientific" Is Science?

As Larry Dossey (1982) observes, "Although science demands proof that observations made by one observer be observable by other observers using the same methods, it is by no means clear that, even when confronted with identical phenomena, different observers will report identical observations" (9). If the content of medical science was unaffected by culture, this would not be the case.

When Payer (1989) investigated biomedical practice in Great Britain, Germany, France, and the United States, she found many differences. The British prescribe fewer drugs in general than the French or Germans. The patient in Great Britain is about one-half as likely as an American to have surgery of any kind. Daily vitamin requirements are smaller. British doctors are more reluctant than American ones to diagnose someone as "sick" based upon similar signs and symptoms.

In Germany, low blood pressure is a condition requiring treatment to raise it, unlike the United States where it is treated as a "nondisease," indicative of long life. Germans prescribe far fewer antibiotics and far more heart drugs than the other nationalities, and they consider the heart to be greatly affected by emotions, rather than a pump that can be replaced.

French biomedicine concentrates on building up the physical and mental constitution (termed "terrain") with vitamins, tonics, diet, and exercise, rather than aggressively attacking the disease with drugs and medications. The French perform very few hysterectomies compared to the United States. Treatment for psychiatric problems is likely to be a visit to a government approved spa, a long sick leave, or a "sleep cure."

Finally, the practice of scientific medicine in the United States is highly aggressive and directed toward attacking the lesion, or disease; the body is considered a machine to be "fixed." As Janet Malcomb noted, even psychoanalysis in the United States is not concerned with emotions, but "rearranges things inside the mind the way surgery rearranges things inside the body" (quoted in Payer 1989: 150). Payer adds that "Anything that cannot fit into the machine model of the body, or be quantified, is often denied not only quantification, but even existence" (151).

These major differences in perception and use of biomedical knowledge and content can be seen to reflect basic cultural values. The French highly value having children and the aesthetics of appearance. The Germans, although characterized as authoritarian, are influenced by nineteenth-century Romanticism and see themselves as emotional, accommodating the various facets of efficiency, spirituality, and nature—hence the focus on the heart. The British practice an "economy" in their medicine, partly due to the payment incentives for doctors, but also because, it is suggested, the British are taught to deny the body. They are expected to exhibit stoicism and maintain a "stiff upper lip" (Payer 1989).

In the United States, the practice of an aggressive, heroic style of biomedicine, where doing something is always better than doing nothing, fits well into the national psyche (mind-set or direction of thinking). The compatibility of heroic medicine with American values was noted by Oliver Wendell Holmes, who wrote:

How could a people . . . which insists in sending out yachts and horses and boys to out-sail, out-run, out-fight, and checkmate all the rest of creation; how could such a people be content with any but 'heroic' practice? What wonder that the Stars and Stripes wave over doses of ninety grains of sulphate of quinine, or that the American eagle screams with delight to see three drachms of calomel given at a single mouthful? (Holmes 1888 [1861]: 193).

These early values and approaches are still dominant. Some treatment decisions have become even more "heroic" with the growth of technological possibilities, such as keeping comatose people alive on respirators;

when there is no hope of recovery or even improvement, such treatment may be interpreted as totally inappropriate (A. Johnson 1996: 20).

The meanings of scientific findings are hotly debated by physicians and scientists alike as they attempt to understand and interpret medical information, using their educational and experiential resources that must include cultural factors of which they may be totally unaware. Some recent cases in point involve how to treat breast cancer and whether the removal of the entire breast with underlying muscle is the best approach; or heart disease and whether more expensive and dangerous bypass surgery is better than less invasive angioplasty, which widens arteries, or even just diet and exercise; and whether or not to treat depression with strong and sometimes dangerous medications with unknown side effects.

The use of synthetic estrogen, for example, was found to be a valid treatment not only for menopausal symptoms, but for prevention of osteoporosis, a degeneration of the bones from loss of natural estrogen after menopause, and for protection against heart disease. Several studies in 1975, however, linked use of estrogen replacement therapy with increased risk of endometrial cancer, and prescriptions declined. Women became uncertain whether or not to undergo the therapy, and doctors were uncertain whether or not to prescribe it (Lock 1993).

Both doctor and patient are dealing with odds and a cost-benefit problem, making absolute decisions based on relative perspectives (Lock 1993: 337–40; Mack and Ross 1989). To the physician, the risk may be worth the benefit, but to the patient, it may not—or vice versa. Therefore, these decisions must be based upon personal and cultural meanings and implications as well as being based on whatever scientific information is available, as interpreted by the physician and considered by the patient.

The problem is compounded because scientific results may also be confusing and subject to different interpretations. For example, Mack and Ross (1989), after performing an extensive risk-benefit analysis of estrogen use (discussed by Lock 1993), recommended "prudent" use of estrogen without other hormones. Most physicians, however, recommend that combined therapy should always be used (reported in Coney 1994). As Dossey observes, "The problem now in medicine is that the fit of the medical model and the clinical observations that physicians actually make are so discrepant as to be beyond salvage" (1982: 10). A major difficulty here is that biomedicine operates within its own cultural constructs and constraints.

BIOMEDICINE AS CULTURE

As opposed to being considered a culture-free system, biomedicine, as we have seen, may be viewed as one element or approach within a larger cultural system. It may also be examined as a cultural system itself (Hahn 1995). One way of characterizing a medical system would be to include the elements of illness, people, environment, resources, and beliefs (Gesler 1991: 21). A medical system would include types of illness present; socially sanctioned healers and the means, method, and content of their training; a structured means of delivery of care; designated locations for care delivery; a means of financing or paying for care; philosophies and ideas about health and illness; and all the links, interactions, inputs, and outputs between and among elements (Robertson and Heagarty 1975). These elements can also be broken down according to their characteristics and vary from medical system to medical system, time, and place. The interrelationships of elements, however, are directed to the purpose of prevention, cure, and control of illness.

The system of biologically based medical care involves a technical language, a central belief and value system, rituals, and symbols different from those of the general society. A. Johnson (1996) refers to this as a "medical paradigm" (a model), which can be compared to other medical paradigms such as that of Hippocrates (18). There can be many variations within the paradigmatic structure. The doctor-patient relationship, for example, may vary according to patient population, setting of care, medical diagnosis, and so forth, and some physicians may be more oriented within the biological, psychological, or social perspectives.

The special language of biomedicine gives clinical meaning to disease through labeling. A diagnosis of infection with *Clostridium tetani*, or tetanus, for example, indicates to the physician that a deep puncture wound allowed anaerobic bacteria to enter the bloodstream of the patient; the tetanospasmin in the toxin binds to the ganglioside membranes of nerve synapses, blocking the release of the inhibitory transmitter from the nerve terminals, thereby causing a generalized tonic spasticity upon which intermittent tonic convulsions are usually superimposed (*The Merck Manual* 1982: 113–14). This, of course, means little or nothing to the patient who suffers and whose ideas of cause and effect may be quite different and include anything from punishment for past sins to plain bad luck.

In many instances, the language of biomedicine is inadequate for discussing various conditions. In discussing Arthur Kleinman's work on suffering (Kleinman 1986b), Shweder notes that suffering comes in many forms and varies across cultures and historical epochs. He points out that Kleinman's work presents a more holistic view of the experience of suffering as caused by loss, defeat, and social injustice, in contrast to causes located within the body (1991: 313). The discourse of our biomedical culture (for example, the disease concept) is thus ill-suited for representing and comprehending some major forms of human suffering (331).

The Extension of Medical Culture and Social Control

The label of "disease," which implies submission to the official medical system designed to address it (Parsons 1951), may not be adequate in addressing suffering. But it has been increasingly applied to a number of human conditions and behaviors defined as **deviant** (i.e., different or apart from the norm).

Since deviance may generally be seen as willful or unwillful, crime and illness may be viewed as alternate designations for deviance (Conrad and Schneider 1992: 36). Deviance not viewed as willful is seen as amenable to help and treatment, rather than as criminal behavior to be punished. Through the process of **medicalization**, physicians define in medical terms what may have been considered a personal or social problem and propose medical treatment as an appropriate solution. When illness is the designation, medicine becomes the agent of social control. In the case of chemical dependency, for example, "medicine replaces or collaborates with the criminal justice system" (P. Brown 1995: 41).

Alcoholism provides a good example. As a medical problem, alcoholism is labeled a disease over which the sufferer has little or no control and is treated with medications and even personal psychiatric counseling, often at inpatient alcohol treatment facilities. Demedicalization would occur when the problem is once again viewed as personal deviance or human weakness to be addressed by education or strong social sanctions and possibly incarceration as punishment.

Other medicalized areas include childbirth (discussed in chapter 3), behavioral manifestations such as hyperactivity and aggressiveness, sleep disorders, and even male baldness. One example of an historical medicalized condition would be women's enjoyment of sexuality. In some places during the nineteenth century, such enjoyment was labeled a disease and was treated, sometimes by even removing the clitoris. Today in some cultures, due to the changing view of women as full participants in society, with a right to recognize the sexual side of their nature, it is considered unhealthy if a woman fails to enjoy her sexuality (A. Johnson 1996). She may now be treated with hormones or counseling for "frigidity" in order to regain her "sexual potential."

Current U.S. culture is quite receptive to the process of medicalization. Capitalism allows for the creation of new and highly profitable markets, and medicalization has the potential for creating new markets through expanded definitions of social and personal problems. Thus, the medical conceptions of deviance in American society have "a cultural resonance both with dominant values and the organizational apparatus to promote and sustain them, creating a fertile environment for medicalization" (Conrad and Schneider 1992: 265).

It is doubtful that the process of medicalization could occur to the extent identified if the appeal were not related to cultural values and norms. For example, drinking has generally been tacitly accepted in our society, particularly among males. It has also been viewed as a norm, a symbol of sociability, recreation, and escape from the stresses of life. "Holding one's liquor" has also been a mark of masculinity. Once a drinker has progressed to the point of becoming an alcoholic, medicalization relieves the drinker of personal responsibility and provides a socially acceptable therapy for recovery. The label makes the problem less devastating for both the drinker and her or his family.

The appeal of medically preventing, halting, or reversing hair loss in males, which is not a medical problem in itself, can be seen as relating to high social values placed on youth. Loss of hair signifies the process of aging and loss of currently defined physical attractiveness. Hair loss as a medical problem can be addressed by medical treatment. Recall the advertisements to "see your doctor" because "there *is* hope," sponsored by a pharmaceutical producer of a drug to stimulate new hair growth. The tenor of the appeal is that of curing a disease condition rather than as a cosmetic appeal to vanity, which in American culture is as unmanly as a receding hairline.

The social sciences have produced numerous attacks on this extension of medical labeling. The medicalization of American society is interpreted as a type of "medical imperialism" that extends medical authority and power over wider aspects of American life (cf. Conrad and Schneider 1992). The invasion of medicine into everyday life, as it is perceived, may compromise the individual's autonomy through overreliance on experts, with loss of abilities to cope (Zola 1972); create a real danger to health in overreliance on medicine, resulting in **iatrogenic** (doctor caused) illnesses (Illich 1976); and be used by the state to maintain the status quo and to suppress particular social groups (Navarro 1976; Waitzkin 1983; Krause 1977).

However, the idea of treatment for alcoholics to help them return to functional social roles, for example, seems both humane and logical. In addition, as seen in both medical sociology and anthropology, the medicalization of problem drinking actually can lead to the investigation into the deeper sources of the problem beyond individual experience, which includes the social structure. For example, Merrill Singer and colleagues, in investigating the seemingly self-destructive drinking behavior of a Puerto Rican subject, revealed the need for a thorough analysis of the wider interpretation of alcoholism as being a "disease of the world economic system, and at the same time, an expression of human suffering and coping, as well as resistance to the forces and pressures of that system" (1992: 100).

Recent social constructivist analyses of the social control function of medicalization characterize social control as a creative force rather than a means of suppression (Armstrong 1989). For example, at the end of the eighteenth century, the body was objectified by viewing it as a machine to be "fixed." At this point, the focus was on the body as a physical entity. Armstrong (1989) argues that this focus was a necessary precedent to later expanding the twentieth-century medical perception of the body into a whole person.

The debate over medicalization will continue, but various intervening social and cultural forces will undoubtedly influence and determine the directions and extent of medical control. As Armstrong (1989) points out, "the future of medicine in its various forms can only be analysed in the context of a society of which it is part, and with which it has reciprocal relations" (130).

Doctor-Patient, Provider-Consumer

The physician, says Hahn, is the center of the biomedical culture (1995). The physician's relationship with the patient is, then, the central element, the focus of the medical care system (Glass 1996). This relationship has long been a topic of study for both medical sociology and anthropology, and includes factors of trust, communication, decision-making, and power.

According to the cultural ideals of biomedicine, the physician possesses the technical abilities, within limits, of alleviating the patient's suffering, treating illness, and preserving life. The patient, on the other hand, is threatened with pain, disability, and the possible end of existence and must rely on the doctor's knowledge, skill, and moral and ethical behavior; this requires a great deal of trust on the part of the patient. That trust has not always been easily established.

There are numerous historical examples of physicians withholding diagnostic information from patients and divulging as little information on patients' conditions as considered possible or prudent (Laine and Davidoff 1996: 152). Even Hippocrates advised concealing information from patients. The rationale included the lack of knowledge on the part of patients, as well as their inability to understand or interpret medical information. This rationale has not entirely disappeared today, but numerous social forces have altered the attitudes and approaches for doctor-patient communication. Better educated patients, the wealth of medical and health care information available to the public, increasing interest in and practice of self-care, the growing problems of chronic illness, the growth and use of technological means of diagnosis and treatment—all have created pressures for change and a more "patient-centered" medicine.

A number of models for the doctor-patient relationship have been identified. Some physicians practice all models at any one time, while others may favor only one or two. The range of models depicts the changing character of the doctor-patient relationship and the move from doctor control to patient-centered medicine. For example, depending upon the severity of the illness, Szasz and Hollender (1956) identified the activity-passivity model, where patients are comatose or otherwise unable to take any active part in their case or where patients are entirely passive to the physician's care; the guidance-cooperation model, where patients may have infectious or acute conditions and cooperate with the decisions of the physician; and the mutual participation model, which was suggested as applicable to "select patients" (i.e., those with greater intellect, education, and experience), but which also appropriately applies to those with chronic conditions where the patient must work with the doctor as a full participant in his or her own care. Szasz and Hollender's suggestion that "guidance-cooperation" was replacing the older "activity-passivity" model seemed almost heretical at the time it was proposed (Laine and Davidoff 1996: 153).

In 1992, Emanuel and Emanuel proposed the paternalistic, informative, interpretive, and deliberative models. Although the authors pointed out that under different clinical conditions, one or the other model might be appropriate, the deliberative model represented the optimal doctor-patient relationship. Both parties would engage in active discourse, which would include the patient's values, perspective, and agreement in treatment decisions. The physician would promote health-related values (e.g., safer sex), but would fit therapies into the patient's cultural frame of reference.

Quill (1983) also saw the ideal doctor-patient relationship as consensual and not obligatory. The relationship becomes contractual, with mutually unique obligations and responsibilities and with decisions reached through negotiation for mutual benefit.

Although models appear to be evolving into an optimal interactive relationship, one model does not necessarily "fit all." Patients from different ethnic groups, for example, often have different attitudes and expectations about patient autonomy. It is also important to remember that ethnicity is not the only indicator of differing needs and expectations. Even previous experience may determine patient preferences.

In their own experiences with migraine headaches, a chronic condition highly resistant to standard treatment and requiring individual management and interpretation, Macintyre and Oldman (1977) point out that while their knowledge of migraines was largely gleaned from medical sources, they felt that their own interpretation of their condition was superior to that of individual doctors (69). Migraine tends to be a highly individual and personal condition that does not neatly fit within any pathological or clinical interpretation. This difference impacts on the doctor-patient relationship, they contend, since their own experience may conflict with what the doctor "knows." They visit their doctor only because the doctor controls access to resources that they need and desire. In this situation, they refuse to adopt the patient role and resent the efforts of the doctor to explore the psychological or social aspects of their problem. They themselves know what helps and what does not, based on experience.

Macintyre and Oldman offer a very different perspective when they note that "Patients have also complained that doctors treat them as 'conditions' or 'objects' rather than as complete persons. Our experience suggests that this is precisely what we want from our doctors. . . . We suspect that, contrary to the views of many 'humanitarian' medical sociologists, many other sufferers of other complaints similarly wish to be treated as a 'case of X' rather than as a 'person' " (1977: 70).

The shift to **patient-centered care**, described by Laine and Davidoff (1996), deemphasizes the idea of compliance and stresses participation; it does, however, allow for some diversity and selectivity in assessing what patients really prefer or want to know. Patients coming from other cultural backgrounds may not expect or even want detailed medical information about their conditions. For example, in Japan that information is commonly withheld.

A series of letters in the *Journal of the American Medical Association* (*JAMA* 1996: 107–10) focused on the Navajo concept of *hózhó*, which prohibits speaking directly of negative issues such as possible complications of surgery, adverse effects of medication, or even death, since to do so makes them more likely to happen. Responses to the difficulty included comments that "refusing to give them the facts about their condition and possible treatment because they belong to a particular ethnic group is not only unethical but absurd" (1996: 108). But they also included suggestions from practitioners who treat Navajo patients and find that use of third-person plural in discussions works very well and that "in general, Navajo patients quickly identify this good faith effort made by the practitioner and seem to be more willing and able to understand the 'negatives' in medicine." This view also recognizes that "Such culturally sensitive communication can lead to more informed decisions and better outcomes" (108). Thus a more patient-centered approach would seem, by definition, to consider the issues of cultural sensitivity and patient expectations and preferences as part of patients' rights.

The conflict over the Navajo case is not an isolated one. Citing the growing tensions between the medical science and medical art (care), including strain due to rapid changes in practice economics such as specialization and technological advance, Glass (1996) states that "The patient-physician relationship is under siege" (147). He notes the narrow focus on the biomedical model, which ignores the important psychosocial factors and isolates physicians from their patients as people. Doctors no longer "listen" to patients, which is vital to the art of medicine. In the old days, before the increase in focus on scientific therapeutics, doctors were encouraged to let the patient talk as a means of therapeutic intervention and included the doctor's respectful and undivided attention, rather than "interrogation" (Shorter 1985: 157–64).

Glass cites a "new paradigm" of **evidence-based medicine**, which emphasizes the critical assessment of clinical science in diagnosis and points out that if the "critical" is emphasized then science need not separate doctor and patient. Physicians should use the best that science has to offer, but not at the expense of an acknowledgment of psychosocial issues or the uniqueness of each patient as a person. However, this view stresses consideration, empathy, and compassion while still being located well within the biomedical paradigm; it does not broaden the "evidence" to include the sociocultural issues outside the biomedical culture that are so vital to communication and understanding.

The strain of health care economics also threatens to intervene in the doctor-patient relationship because of the intensifying problems of need and cost inherent in exchange of fee-for-service. With the recent direct entry of corporate entities into the health care field, the discourse of medicine has begun to take on the language of the market place. Patients become "clients" or "consumers," physicians become "providers." Incentives change as medical care becomes a "product" to be purchased. Major concerns cited by Glass include less time spent with each patient, loss of physician autonomy in clinical decision-making, loss of continuity in patient care, loss of patient trust, and the adversarial and ethical problems that arise when decisions are driven by financial concerns rather than by the best interests of the patient (1996: 1296).

The trend toward patient-centered care may prove to offset some of the negative influences of marketplace medicine. Paradoxically, this trend may actually be supported by consumerism, since new consumers of health care are more informed, wish to have their own preferences considered, and have become more accustomed to questioning physician authority (Laine and Davidoff 1996). Patient-centered care may also help address the problem of malpractice suits against physicians since it has been shown that various physician behavior such as disrespect and devaluing or ignoring patients' questions and perspectives are positively associated with malpractice claims (Laine and Davidoff 1996; also see Beckman et al. 1994).

Again paradoxically, corporate focus on the bottom line may ultimately serve to bring doctors and patients back together. In the role of patient advocate, physicians may join with patients to "hold third parties accountable to their claims that high quality of care, rather than purely low cost, is their mission" (Laine and Davidoff 1996: 155). In support of that possibility, *JAMA* (the AMA's journal) has initiated a new section specifically dealing with patient-centered care. The base of biomedical knowledge may be expanded to include social implications and the perspectives and concerns of patients.

One final note on patient-centered care relates to the previously discussed need to consider patients as part of a family or household unit (see chapter 2) that is directly affected by the illness of any of its members. It must also be remembered that patient-centered care is in reality "family-centered care" and that the doctor-patient dyad must be expanded to include family and household members. This inclusion and consideration of individual and family wants, needs, and rights has become, along with other issues in medical practice, a matter of moral and ethical concern.

BIOETHICS IN CULTURAL CONTEXT

Although social scientists do not all agree on what constitutes a profession, having a code of ethics is one criteria. The American biomedical profession's ethical stance on right or wrong conduct in research and patient care reflects the need to consider the welfare of patients. The perception and definition of patient welfare, however, may vary.

Codified or not, ethical decision-making has always been a part of the profession of biomedicine, whether those decisions were made jointly by patients and doctors, doctors alone, or as accepted policies in health care institutions. Early Western medical ethics were reflected, in part, in the Hippocratic oath, which exhorts physicians, if they cannot help, to at least "do no harm." Ethics were located within the context of possibilities (i.e., existing knowledge and the boundaries of the physician's role). The moral exhortation to "do no harm" recognizes that harm is certainly possible. As previously noted, the service versus profit orientation was also recognized from early on, along with its temptations and possibilities. Ethical codes, then, not only can be a measure of professionalism, but can serve as a means of social control over "unethical behavior," using the threat of loss of professional identity and status.

With the greater capacities of modern medicine to do good, the potential to do harm is also increased, even when unintentional. "Harm" is not an easy concept to define, in view of the fact that medicine must often harm in order to heal, as in the case of chemotherapy for cancer. Also, what is harm to one may not be harm to another, as in invasive or painful treatment to maintain life when no benefit or improvement can be derived.

Bioethics (ethics applied to biomedicine) as part of biomedicine also cannot be viewed as acultural or outside of the influences of cultural considerations. The main stuff of bioethics concerns human values and beliefs that reflect or are translated into social structure and activity.

Bioethical debates are being conducted in an increasingly pluralistic, culturally fragmented, and "religiously resonant but secularized society" (Fox 1994: 49). In this atmosphere, many feel the need for and therefore support a simplified, common, and broadly applicable way of addressing moral and ethical problems; thus, ethical issues are generally located (and generated) within the framework of the dominant culture. The ethical principles to be applied are also located within that framework and conform to a paradigm of "principlism," which derives from an "Anglo-American analytic and secular philosophical tradition" (McCormick 1994). The bioethical agenda, in other words, "responds to the predominating political, economic, and value orientation of the society, which tends to reflect rather than criticize or challenge" and is more "reactive than initiatory" (Fox 1994: 49).

Some ethicists and social scientists feel that ethics discussed or considered within this "formulaic" framework have become flat, mechanical, unemotional, and formal (Fox 1994; Gustafson 1990). Such discussions are also devoid of any recognition of cultural needs and diversity. Attempts by both sociologists and anthropologists to apply cultural sensitivity to research on the subject by recognizing and respecting cultural diversity have been criticized as essentially irrelevant and "no substitute for careful moral analysis" (Ijsselmuiden and Faden 1992: 833).

Multiculturalism presents a substantial challenge to bioethics, because cultural values and ethical frameworks are often in conflict. Respect for individual autonomy for example, is a basic principle of Western bioethics. In many cultures, however, such as some Asian or Hispanic groups, family, community, and interdependence are much more important than individual autonomy.

As an ethical issue, the question of abortion also becomes highly complex when viewed cross-culturally. The concepts of "human" and "person" are quite distinct in many non-Western societies. The rights accorded to persons may be quite different from those accorded to humans. In some societies, after biological birth, a fetus (still so regarded by the community) must earn the status and rights of "person" by managing to survive, gaining the vigor and health necessary for becoming a contributing member of the community; it then experiences a "social birth," which confers the rights of personhood (Morgan 1989). Most societies condemn infanticide, but only after the neonate has been recognized as a person. And as Morgan explains, "The social construction of personhood differs according to the environmental, cosmological, and historical circumstances of different societies. . . . There can be no absolute definition of personhood isolated from a sociocultural context" (101).

Further difficulty in developing multicultural bioethics is created by the capitalist context: bioethics, like other elements of the dominant medical system, have been subject to marketplace discourse. There is discussion of cost containment, competition, health care as a commodity subject to supply and demand, allocation of resources, economic returns from research investments, the body as private property, and questions of supply and demand for organ transplantation.

Framing bioethical issues in terms of profit and loss leads away from a service orientation or one that considers health care as a social good; "furthermore, it removes the field from a conception of social justice that pays special attention to the plight of the poor, the disadvantaged, the victims of social prejudice and discrimination" (Fox 1994: 50). The service orientation, on the other hand, establishes the relevance and connection of medical ethical issues with sociostructural causes of illness and with social injustice, which includes unequal access to health care for many groups.

Although consideration of costs and benefits seems to conflict with ethical considerations, when many people are left out of the system due to high costs and the inability to pay, economic problems must be addressed as a subject of ethical concern. In addition, in an age of legal tangles and multiple interpretations, Supreme Court decisions, uncertainty, and fear of lawsuits—as well as confusion, human anguish, and unwillingness and inability to confront hard choices—there is a need for guidelines and the creation of some precedents, as well as recognition that resources and capabilities are finite.

Medical ethics (or bioethics) has become a respected area of expertise, with a number of established centers throughout the United States. Bioethics is a uniquely human endeavor—and as such, it must reflect the diversity of human needs and perceptions. While experts can study the problems and issues and give advice and consultation, they, too, may have vested interests and agendas; they may "know" but not "see" (Lieberman 1970). Experts may determine policies and options for decision-making and recommend courses of action, but the possible risks and benefits for individuals must also be assessed by the one most affected—the patient—or, when this is not possible, by those who can best represent him or her. To this end, bioethics committees, composed of both professional experts and lay participants, are seen as a most desirable option for consultation, reviewing cases, and offering advice to be taken or rejected by the patient or parties involved (Munson 1996).

The field of bioethics faces the same problems of the need for respect for diversity as those faced in biomedicine and society in general. It must allow for a broader, more inclusive view of human needs and emotions while maintaining a sense of unity in ethical guidelines and recognition of the human condition. The same is true for the biomedical model.

EXPANDING THE BIOMEDICAL MODEL

Nursing's Sunrise Model

The Sunrise Model, conceived and constructed by Madelaine Leininger, a registered nurse who has done doctoral work in anthropology, is a strong indicator of the involvement and participation of the field of nursing in the forefront of promoting cultural sensitivity in medicine and medical care.

Developing her model in the 1970s, Leininger recognized that people differ culturally in the ways they view professional nursing and client care needs. She was aware that cultural factors influence client behavior, as well as well-being and outcome of care, and recognized the related need for nurses to consider both the emic (local) and etic (in this case, science's) views in treating and caring for their patients. She also distinguished between humanistic caring and scientific caring—relating the first to subjective feelings, experiences, and interactions, and the second to those activities and judgments that have been tested or are based on verified and quantified knowledge related to specific variables.

Nurses, although trained within the scientific biomedical paradigm, have long recognized both the needs and benefits of a dual approach, since they are the providers who deal most continuously with the pain and suffering of patients in their care. The Sunrise Model reflects holistic facets and dimensions of caring for patients in a culturally sensitive way and highlights "world view, religion, kinship, cultural values, economics, technology, language, ethnohistory, and environmental factors that are predicted to explain and influence culture care" (Leininger 1993: 26–27).

At the same time that nursing has become and is becoming more professionalized and subject to the same commercializing forces as those faced by physicians, Leininger's idea of "culture care" might be seen as a reaction to the deemphasis and loss of the focus on caring in the health professions. Although certainly most applicable in nursing, the lessons of culture care are relevant to the medical profession, to physicians, and to all who provide care to the ill and suffering.

Holistic Health

Holistic health, which has developed as a movement within the last two decades, presents an alternative medical paradigm with a different arrangement of medical practice and patient-practitioner relationships. It also offers some possibilities for consideration in biomedical practice.

Holistic practitioners constitute a highly varied and diverse group, ranging from faith healers, chiropractors, and herbalists to mainstream physicians who may use some holistic techniques. Lowenberg (1989), however, derived seven core beliefs that holistic practitioners hold in common. Generally, they view the person as a whole being situated within a total environment and see health promotion and education as vital to the healing process. The meaning of illness to holistic adherents involves all aspects of the client—including the mental, emotional, social, spiritual, and physical.

The individual, if able, takes much responsibility for understanding his or her own illness, initiating steps to prevent illness and promote health, and actively participates in treatment. Practitioners, rather than taking the role of expert as biomedical practitioners do, become facilitators, educators, and consultants, sharing expertise with more self-directed clients. There is ideally a warm, caring setting for care delivery and more physical contact between patient and practitioner, which is seen as an important component in healing (Krieger 1984).

The last characteristic concerns an alternative world view, or view of "consciousness." The focus on consciousness might be considered a shift of paradigms—from a reductionist, objectivist model to a more all-inclusive world view related to the nature of reality. This shift is sometimes compared to the shift from Newtonian to quantum physics (Dossey 1982).

As an alternative medical model, holism is most likely to offer elements and ideas for incorporation into the dominant medical paradigm, filling gaps and providing alternative explanations for problems not addressed by the biomedical model. Nevertheless, the holistic model itself also contains a number of problems and limitations that must be recognized—particularly in the area of self-responsibility and doctor-patient relationships.

Making the individual primarily responsible for his or her own health and illness puts the patient in charge, but also reinforces the attitude of "blaming the victim" when an individual becomes ill. It can also be lethal. One 44-year-old female college professor with malignant melanoma, a deadly skin cancer, tried mental imagery to effect a cure, but "when it failed to arrest the disease, she began to blame herself. 'She was pained by the possibility that her own psychological defects brought on the disease and precluded her ability to cure herself' " (Cassileth, cited in G. Williams 1993: 78).

Dossey cautions that the holistic insistence on the concept of individual self is inconsistent with the true meaning of the term, which involves an interconnection with all other individuals and environments. "The holistic movement," notes Dossey, "commits the same failure as the traditional system of medical care by placing primacy on the *objectivity* of health care" and both paradigms are still located in a similar world view of cause and effect (Dossey 1982: 214, italics in original).

Similarities between the holistic and the biomedical model also are suggested by Berliner and Salmon (1980) in patterns of fee-for-service entrepreneurial practice, knowledge sold to consumers as a commodity, elitist and sexist behavior of practitioners, availability of services to middle-class clients and those who can pay, clear separation between clients and practitioners, and total disregard of larger societal factors as causing and contributing to disease (143).

Research on outcomes of holistic treatment has often been contradictory and inconclusive (Watkins 1996: 55–57). Incorporation and integration with biomedical treatments would seem to hold the most promise, but much more research on outcomes of holistic approaches alone, in contrast to, and in combination with biomedical therapies is needed. If this is to take place, however, Watkins notes that "these systems either have to be proven effective by allopathic [biomedical] mechanisms, or allopathy has to accept that *they may work via mechanisms that are foreign to the present biomedical model*" (emphasis added) (1996: 55).

The Biopsychosocial Model

In response to the reductionist biomedical model, George Engel (1977) advanced a new model that would be inclusive of the other personal dimensions of which the physical is only a part: the **biopsychosocial model**. The actual impetus for the generation of this model came from within medicine itself, and its construction was a recognition that in order to provide effective medical care, the psychosocial factors would have to be addressed. Engel's model appeared originally as a "psychiatric" perspective with the ultimate goal of integration into all biomedical education (Lyng 1990).

Engel (1977) recognized a tremendous advantage in the biomedical approach, but also saw the limitations that were reflected in public dissatisfaction with the growing dehumanization apparent in biomedical practice, as well as a multitude of problems such as unnecessary hospitalization, an overuse of drugs and medications, unnecessary surgery, and inappropriate diagnostic testing (134). The biopsychosocial model was also constructed on the basis of systems theory. It provided a framework, an integrated hierarchy, for the separate domains of health—the biological, psychological, and social—as a means of identifying their relationships and, thereby, the holistic nature of medicine.

Engel recognized that social factors could influence the existence and perceptions of disease; however, he still accorded biomedicine the top status in the hierarchy and advocated the inclusion of the psychosocial dimensions of illness, "soundly based on scientific principles" (1977: 135). Therefore, rather than providing an inclusive model, the biopsychosocial model essentially co-opts the psychosocial under the bio. Systems theory neutralizes the challenges of alternatives by simply presenting them as different levels of explanation of the same phenomena, thus they remain compatible with the biomedical model (Armstrong 1987: 1214). The reductionist model of biomedicine and the primacy of science is thus not only maintained, but is strengthened.

The "new model," argues Armstrong, is "simply the old one with a gloss" (1987: 1217). In addition, Armstrong cites the sociological research of recent years that challenges many of the assumptions of science and the biomedical perspective, that is, the statistical definition of "normal" and "proper functioning," the social definitions and concepts of disease, and the social, economic, and political influences that played a large part in the rise of biomedical dominance, all of which are ignored by Engel.

From Armstrong's perspective, the biopsychosocial model will neither deconstruct nor reconstruct the world of illness. On the other hand, the model might provide a means to shift the biomedical perspective. It has opened the door to consideration of psychological and social dimensions of the patient as a person. If, for example, in conjunction with other growing expressions of the limitations of a biomedical approach, the biopsychosocial model encourages exploration of alternative structures and possibilities, it can provide an expansion, rather than a confirmation, of the reductionist model. It may have already done so.

The Need for a Multicultural Orientation

Although for some people, both within and outside of the health care professions, the idea of the need for cultural understanding and sensitivity in health care is still a controversial issue, from a practical and professional perspective, the practice of medicine is, by nature, multicultural. Where the culture of biomedicine comes into contact with other medicines and other cultures, it is also syncretic. Each may learn from the other, with adaptations and incorporation of techniques and philosophies. But this requires communication and mutual respect.

Biomedicine, as a service-oriented profession dedicated to the alleviation of suffering for people of all cultures, has a responsibility to reexamine its own motivations, goals, and ethical ideals in the pursuit of that goal. Cure must be reconciled with care, and care must be conceptualized in ways consistent with patient perceptions. In the next chapter, we discuss a number of ways that medical care providers can become more culturally sensitive in order to enhance both their curing and their caring.

FOR DISCUSSION

1. Discuss early medical care in the United States. How did it reflect medical pluralism and a multicultural population?

2. What factors, other than scientific advances, have contributed to the development of the American biomedical system? How could we characterize the American biomedical system in terms of its consistency with the dominant culture?

3. What are some of the difficulties and challenges faced by the American biomedical system today? Consider the various social, cultural, and economic changes taking place in the United States. What predictions might we make as to future evolution and development?

4. Discuss the values and limitations of possible new models of health care. What type of model would be most useful and reasonable, and how could it be promoted and implemented? Can the orientations of profit and public service be compatible?

6

Gathering and Interpreting Cultural Information: The Communication of Meaning

> When we think of all [the] tasks in the consultation, what is surprising is not
> how often we fail, but that we ever succeed.... Even when patients and
> doctors come from a common culture, neither participant has any idea what
> the other is talking about much of the time.... In one sense, every consul-
> tation can be thought of as a cross-cultural one.
>
> [Fuller and Toon 1988: 27–28]

Goal: To comprehend the possible dangers of assuming that, even when
the same language is spoken, communication between patient and practitioner is non-problematic; to understand the range of potential barriers to
verbal and nonverbal communication.

Goal: To acquire some of the background needed for gaining knowledge
of client needs, satisfaction, or health knowledge and practices.

Because of the disease orientation of biomedicine and the tendency to
medicalize or reduce problems to the organic level, recommendations for
diagnosis and treatment within the biomedical system did not, until recently, begin to include the consideration of cultural beliefs, values, or practices. The great impact these have on health and illness has long been
demonstrated by social scientists and is now being acknowledged by some
biomedical professionals (e.g., Eisenberg and Kleinman 1981; Helman
1995).

The nursing profession has for some time promoted the benefits of "culture care" (Leininger 1985), but many physicians may still resist the suggestion that they address a patient's emotional and psychological needs as

well as his or her physiological problems, and they may not see the benefits of doing so. As one physician commented to Loustaunau in a personal discussion, "Do you mean to tell me that when I'm trying to treat a patient or save a life, I should be considering their cultural values and attitudes? That is utterly absurd!"

This attitude reflects the reductionist model of medical care and totally excludes the role of social and psychological factors in health and illness. It is true that physicians and other health care providers may also be concerned that being culturally sensitive entails a great deal of extra study, effort, and time that they do not have. But considering the multicultural nature of the U.S. population and the projections for increasing multiculturalization, it becomes imperative for clinicians with a service orientation to all people who are ill, suffering, or in pain to apply both the science and art of medicine in the cause of healing (Kreps and Kunimoto 1994).

There is a growing body of literature relating to incorporation of cultural assessment into medical care. Although some effort may be required to do this, even at minimal levels the returns can be well worth the investment. Although more research is needed on actual medical outcomes for patients who receive culturally sensitive care and patients who do not, the research that has been done suggests that culturally sensitive care can affect patient compliance, satisfaction, comfort, and attitude toward the medical establishment. Compliance relates strongly to physiological outcome (DiMatteo and DiNicola 1982). Noncompliance may not only endanger the patient's health and well-being, it may increase costs, exacerbate illness, lead to the requirement for further tests and treatment, create discomfort and confusion, produce false or misleading results of clinical research efforts (such as in measuring the effectiveness of a new drug), and jeopardize the patient-practitioner relationship through continual frustration (3).

The increasing prevalence of chronic disease over acute conditions also creates the necessity of patient participation in their own care, which in turn requires trust, respect, and full understanding between physician and patient. Groce and Zola (1993) conclude that "No one individual can anticipate all the problems that might arise in an attempt to understand chronic illness and disability in a multicultural society, but we can all have enough sensitivity to realize that there might be significant differences, and enough respect for others to ask questions and listen carefully to the replies" (1055).

Essentially, practitioners need to be aware that the perceptions clients hold may differ from biomedical ones, and that clients need to be made to feel comfortable if they are to discuss their concerns. Developing the ability to communicate is, therefore, essential. Another strategy for clinicians who would be culturally sensitive is to develop networks of contacts within the communities to be served. And most important of all, they need to develop a sensitivity to health needs as defined by those communities. As Fuller and Toon have noted, "The greater the cultural distance between doctor and patient, the less likely their expectations of the consultation and its outcome are to be congruent" (1988: 27–28).

ISSUES OF COMMUNICATION

The Problem of Compliance

Doctors often become frustrated when patients do not comply with instructions, and it is estimated that over 60 percent of patients who visit biomedical practitioners are to some degree noncompliant (DiMatteo and DiNicola 1982). Clients consulting practitioners generally are offered advice, but they or those who care for them are not generally forced to **comply** with any given regimen. They are given the option to consider and then to act on certain instructions. The reasons for noncompliance are varied, but the rejection of or failure to act on instructions is generally not due to a patient's uncooperative nature or ignorance, as some doctors conclude.

For example, Snow tells of a young first-time mother whose baby was failing to gain weight. After numerous consultations and one hospitalization, the pediatrician recommended a special formula high in calories and nutrients. The mother began to cry. As Snow explains, "A few questions revealed that she had not had enough money to buy formula in the first place and, when told that her baby needed a certain number of ounces/day, she had diluted the bottles to make sure that he got the proper amount" (1993: 245).

Other research reveals similar findings. For example, in his review of the biomedical literature, Schmidt (1978) found that only 20 percent of inner-city children for whom a ten-day course of penicillin was prescribed actually received it. Poverty may certainly have been a factor.

However, financial stress is not the only cause for noncompliance; if it were, we would expect to find total compliance among those with financial resources. But Schmidt also noted that less than 50 percent of "the more comfortable middle class children" were given medicine as prescribed (1978: 308). Factors other than money, such as cultural expectations for consultations or for medication's effects, can influence compliance. Information we have on this subject is limited mostly to biomedical consultations. Whether people comply more or less, and why, to nonbiomedical practitioner recommendations definitely needs further investigation.

Compliance and Intercultural Communication

A reasonable amount of time is necessary for good communication to take place. But communication also requires a number of skills: one must be able to express oneself in a manner understood by others and must be able to listen to and properly interpret information offered and questions asked by others. Previous knowledge and experience can affect the efficacy of both expression and interpretation.

One of the measures of communication is how much information gets transmitted. The need for information rather than treatment may actually be what brings many clients to clinicians. Some go only for a diagnosis. Further, some go only for ailments that are new to them. Others go to make sure a condition is under control or to confirm their own treatment regimen is working (Snow 1993: 129).

However much they may desire information, findings from studies cited in Hahn's 1995 review of the literature on patient-practitioner interaction suggest that one in five patients ask no questions at all and that 13 percent of patient questions go unanswered (169). Patients in one study of biomedical consultations spent an average of only 8 seconds asking questions. Physicians in the study believed that they spend an average of 9 full minutes providing information, when in actuality they spent an average of 1.3 minutes doing so (Waitzkin 1985: 89). Compliance based on maybe 80 seconds worth of information transmission may, by definition, be problematic—especially when patient recall of doctor's explanations and instructions has been reported at only 50 percent (as cited in Hahn 1995: 168).

The work of DiMatteo and DiNicola (1982) on achieving patient compliance focused on the social-psychological aspects of the doctor-patient relationship and the limitations of the biomedical model. Milton Davis (introduction to DiMatteo and DiNicola 1982) pointed out the connections between physical and psychological symptoms and noted that even the patient may not recognize the psychological roots of his or her problems, presenting only physical manifestations: "The very crux of the matter may be overlooked, for in fact between 50 and 75 percent of patients who seek medical care have no positive physical findings—their problems are primarily psychosocial" (xi).

Although a valuable contribution to a complex problem, this approach still fails to consider cultural contexts, as well as social-structural factors that may heavily affect patient compliance. "Compliance" may, in fact, be the wrong term; it implies that people act with totally free wills and ignores the constraints under which we function. As DiMatteo and DiNicola concluded, "A truly ethical approach to compliance enhancement, then, demands the full participation of the patient in both decisions about and implementation of medical treatment" (1982: 276). So a better term may be "mutual cooperation."

The power structure of many biomedical consultations limits the role of the patient, and so do class differences: Waitzkin identified a class-based cultural communication barrier (1985: 98). American working-class patients may tend to communicate more with tone and gesture than directly.

Physicians, who are mainly from middle- and upper-class backgrounds, may be accustomed to direct verbal inquiries and so may fail to hear the nonverbal questions.

Further, people who speak the same language or share the same language base can "talk past" each other. Cultural rules, including rules regarding doctor-patient consultations, are generally implicit or tacit and "each party assumes without discussion that it is their rules that both are using" (Fuller and Toon 1988: 28), even when they are not.

The language of the biomedical culture is grounded in bodies and their mechanics, diagnoses, and repair. But, as seen in chapter 5, the medical lexicon also serves to bind the medical community together and helps its members express the reality of their own lives and experiences; it also distinguishes them from nonmedical personnel and patients.

The use in clinics of the biomedical slang referred to as "medspeak" or "doc talk" and the rationalization by clinicians that communication is not important because patients could not possibly understand medical terminology is another major problem. This bias, as well as a disregard for cultural and personal attitudes, values, beliefs, and concerns, and the insistence by clinicians on total medical control, has worked against the establishment of bonds of trust and, therefore, communication.

Even when clients do have some familiarity with biomedical terminology, miscommunication may occur. Clients and clinicians may use the terminology in different ways (Helman 1995: 139). For example, black people who report having "high blood," "pressure," or "high-pertension" do not refer to the same things that clinicians do when they say "hypertension" or "high blood pressure." First, while the last two terms are the same to clinicians, for Blacks "high-pertension" means increased tension or stress, combined with increased blood volume. Pressure, or "high blood," on the other hand, just means having too much blood or blood that is too high in the body (Heurtin-Roberts and Reisin 1990; Snow 1993: 117–34).

Hypertension, biomedically defined, is something altogether different, so it is important to make sure that when similar terms are used that the meanings attributed also are the same. If not, adherence to clinician suggestions will be poor, and the physician will not address the problem that really concerns the patient.

Using a Translator

People who do not speak the same primary or native language have an even more difficult time communicating in the clinic setting. The most obvious strategy when clinician and client do not speak the same language is to use a translator. But simply finding someone who speaks the same language as the client is not enough. For example, it is important that written material be made available to the client or his or her family, as advice might not be fully remembered after a consultation (and it should not be assumed that people always can read the languages that they speak) (Fuller and Toon 1988: 46–47). It also is essential that instructions given (e.g., how to cleanse a healing wound at home) are given in logical sequence; if x precedes y, then instructions should be stated that way: "Do x and then y" (46).

The translator must be perceived of as nonthreatening and encouraging to the client (Fuller and Toon 1988: 45). Moreover, s/he must be trusted to translate the clinician's communications exactly, without editing or altering what is said. An exception would be in the case of idiomatic expressions, which may not make sense when translated literally into another language. We are reminded of a friend who had a visitor from another country to dinner. Having eaten his fill, the man announced that he was "fed up." While literally this was the case, had the hosts not known more about the man they may have interpreted what he said as aggressive and insulting.

Two more examples help illustrate the problematic nature of idiomatic expressions. Both are taken from Geri-Ann Galanti's U.S. case study collection (1991), as are most of the other examples used in this section. The first example involves a "Chinese-born physician [who] called the night nurse one evening to check on a patient scheduled for surgery the next day. The nurse advised the physician that she noticed a new hesitancy in the patient's attitude. 'To tell you the truth, doctor, I think Mrs. Colby is getting cold feet.' The physician was not familiar with this idiom, suspected circulation problems, and ordered vascular tests" (Galanti 1991: 17).

In a different but similar case, a "nervous patient jokingly asked his surgeon if he was going to 'kick the bucket.' The Korean physician, wanting to reassure the patient that his upcoming surgery would be successful, responded affably, 'Oh, yes, you are definitely going to kick the bucket!' The patient was not reassured" (Galanti 1991: 17).

These examples are doubly significant. Not only do they demonstrate how nonsensical idiomatic expressions can be, but they also show that the linguistically divergent individual need not be the patient. And they show, also, that translation may be happening in an individual's own thoughts and not just through a translator.

Some health care settings have paid translators on call who provide professional and continuous service, resulting in a patient-translator-clinician team that persists for the duration of the treatment. Such continuity is very important (Fuller and Toon 1988: 40). Some clinics even have cross-cultural advocates, "trained members of a particular ethnic group who act as go-betweens for that group and the institution" (37). Advocates interpret but also educate health workers about their cultures and the economic and health problems typical among members of their group. They review health education materials that target their group; assist patients in understanding their options, for example, as in regard to surgery and its implications; and help staff members understand, and thereby reduce, institutional racism (37). Staff members who are not open to constructive criticism of their workplace culture may find this very threatening (38). Unfortunately, they may fear a loss of control in their jobs or take personally criticisms that are meant to improve the system.

Many clinics and hospitals cannot afford this service, let alone professional translators. If a member of the staff speaks a language common to the clients, he or she might be called upon. A friend or relative of the client might also serve as a translator in an emergency.

Despite their best intentions, relatives who volunteer do not always provide good translations. Besides their lack of familiarity with medical terms and procedures (Fuller and Toon 1988: 36), they have other roles to play in relation to the patient, and certain role expectations may conflict with the messages they are asked to relay by clinicians. Moreover, clinicians must think carefully about clients' right to confidentiality, which should not be violated; clients may not wish to reveal certain details in the presence of family or friends (see also Fuller and Toon 1988: 39).

For example, husbands or boyfriends are not always good translators when collecting a woman's reproductive history. The woman may not want her partner to know about past abortions, sexually transmitted diseases (STDs), contraceptive use, or pregnancies. Her concerns about self-presentation and preserving her self-esteem and that of others may override her interest in meeting the clinician's need for accuracy. Talk of reproductive matters between children and parents also can be problematic, as the following example shows.

GRACIELA GARCIA

A Hispanic woman, Graciela Garcia, had to sign an informed consent form for a hysterectomy. Her bilingual son served as the interpreter. When he described the procedure to his mother, he appeared to be translating accurately and indicating the appropriate body parts. His mother signed willingly. The next day, however, when she learned that her uterus had been removed and that she could no longer bear children, she became very angry and threatened to sue the hospital. What went wrong?

Because it is inappropriate for a Hispanic male to discuss her private parts with his mother, the embarrassed son explained that a tumor would be removed from her abdomen and pointed to that general area. When Mrs. Garcia learned that her uterus had been removed, she was quite angry and upset because a Hispanic woman's status is derived in large part from the number of children she produces. (Galanti 1991: 15)

As Galanti notes in discussing this case, "Even speaking the same language is not always sufficient. Cultural rules often dictate who can discuss what with whom" (1991: 16). Another important aspect of this case is the way in which the translator edited for the mother. Editing also can happen in the other direction: some translators will consider themselves representatives of their culture or of the person for whom they are translating, and they will take pains to eliminate any statement that might reflect poorly on the patient or on their group.

NONVERBAL COMMUNICATION

Expressivity

Cultural rules dictate who talks about what, to whom, and also when discussion should take place to begin with, as well as at what pace it should proceed and at what decibel (Kreps and Kunimoto 1994: 116). Members of some cultures tend to be loud and verbally expressive when they wish to demonstrate interest and concern.

Silence is another form of expression, and its value is quite high in some cultures. This can have ramifications for provider-client interaction (see Fuller and Toon 1988: 33–34).

JIM NEZ

Ellen was trying to teach her Navaho patient, Jim Nez, how to live with his newly diagnosed diabetes. She soon became extremely frustrated because she felt she was not getting through to him. He asked very few questions and never met her eyes. She reasoned from this that he was uninterested and therefore not listening to her.

Rather than signaling disinterest, however, Mr. Nez's behavior demonstrated a respect for the nurse's authority. The Navaho value silence. A person who interrupts while someone is speaking is perceived as immature. Most Americans are uncomfortable with silences and tend to fill them with words, making "small" talk. The Navaho use silence to formulate their thoughts. Words should have significance. (Galanti 1991: 16)

Silence may signal respect, but again, it may not—it may reflect fear. A Laotian refugee being treated for stomach cancer refused to talk to a hospital social worker because, says Galanti, she seemed to "have feared that anything she said would have repercussions for her family still in Laos and Thailand" (1991: 28; see also Fuller and Toon 1988: 39). Silence also may signal embarrassment at a lack of command of one's host country's language. In traditional Chinese and Japanese cultures, silence on the part of the speaker signals that s/he wants the listener to consider carefully the content of what s/he said before s/he goes on speaking. A black person may remain silent after being asked a question that s/he perceives as ridiculous. French, Spanish, and Russian people may interpret silence as signaling agreement (Fuller and Toon 1988: 48). Clearly, cultural context and individual acculturation levels must be taken into account when interpreting a silent reaction.

Expressing Pain

Pain is one of the symptoms used by biomedical practitioners in diagnosing illness; it is perceived as a signal that something is wrong. However, classic studies by Zborowski (1952) and Zola (1966) found that cultural ideas about expressiveness and stoicism influenced the expression of pain response for several ethnic groups. Although this knowledge is important, there is a consequent danger of inadvertent stereotyping and false expectations in physicians who treat these patients. Numerous other variables may intervene, such as degree of acculturation, age of patient, educational background, and personal experience. Still, such research shows that to a significant degree, people may be willing to tolerate pain as a function of the expectations of other people. A clinician trained in one culture could easily misinterpret pain expressed in another.

OSITO SEISAY

Some patients tolerate even the most severe pain with little more than a clenched jaw and frequently will refuse pain medication. Osito Seisay, a Nigerian farmer who had been injured by a charging bull, was in the United States for arthro-microscopic knee surgery. His nurse waited for him to request pain medication, but he never did. Mr. Seisay was Muslim, and he offered his pain to Allah in thanks for the good fortune of being allowed such specialized surgery. (Galanti 1991: 25)

MARY CARROLL

[Mary Carroll] was scheduled for surgery at the end of the week. Her family became very concerned when she suddenly started complaining of pain. They knew Mrs. Carroll was typically Irish in her stoicism. They spoke to her doctor, who was from India. He was not worried. In his country, women were usually vocal when in pain. He ignored their requests that the surgery be done sooner, thinking it unnecessary. When he finally did operate, he discovered that Mrs. Carroll's condition had progressed to the point that she could not be saved. (Galanti 1991: 27)

This example makes clear how important it is for medical staff to be culturally aware of the relativity of the expression of pain.

Other Modes of Communication

Eye contact is another mode of communication that can have wide cultural variation. As a part of doctor-patient communication, Shorter (1985) points out that the physician's gaze has often been interpreted as vital and therapeutic in that the eyes of the physician reflect the knowledge and caring that inspire trust and reassurance. The patient gaze, however, is generally not even discussed and may also be read by the physician according to preconceived cultural ideas. When a patient will not meet the doctor's eyes, for example, it could signal shame, prevarication, or anger.

Aversion of the eyes, however, also can signal respect, as in the case of many Asian and West African cultures. Fuller and Toon describe how "an English doctor therefore with a West African patient may feel that she or he is depressed, hostile, or not being straightforward, when in fact there is merely a difference of cultural convention. Conversely, the African patient may experience the English doctor's eye contact as excessive staring" (1988: 51).

Sometimes, eyes are seen as spiritual windows, so direct eye contact can endanger those involved. Other times, direct contact signals intimacy. Or it can signal a sexual invitation. Eye contact with certain patients might be misinterpreted as sexual interest; this can be distressing both for staff members whose patients are convinced they are making advances (Galanti 1991: 17) and for patients who, especially when eye contact is accompanied by what is meant to be reassuring touch, are convinced they are being sexually harassed (Fuller and Toon 1988: 51).

Other forms of **nonverbal communication** that might become important during a consultation include one's physical **proximity** to clients. For instance, while Americans, Canadians, and British people require substantial space between themselves and other people (Gross 1992: 109 reports this at about four feet), Latin Americans, Japanese, and Arabs prefer very little (about two feet for Latin Americans, according to Gross; Fuller and Toon 1988: 51; these researchers caution that most evidence on distance is anecdotal, and recommend further research). Clients may attempt to pull clinicians into—or push them out of—personal space in order to make themselves more comfortable (cf. Fuller and Toon 1988: 51; see also Hall 1980 [1959]).

Habitual **gestures** also must be taken into account; they might have different meanings cross-culturally. While a nod of the head means "yes" to most Americans, Greek and some other Mediterranean people say "no" by a similarly vertical move of the head (Gross 1992: 109; Fuller and Toon 1988: 50). An American clinician might beckon a patient forward by wiggling the index finger out and in with the palm up and other fingers and thumb closed or bent in toward the palm. But this gesture is used in the Philippines to call animals (Galanti 1991: 22). Information on gestures relevant to the population(s) served by one's clinic can help one to avoid embarrassing both oneself and one's clients.

Courtesy and Civility

Courtesy and civility can do much to enhance a relationship and improve communication. However, even this form of expression may be culturally relative. For example, some people may not wish to bother nurses, even when in pain, for to do so would be disrespectful.

A sense of politeness also might lead a patient to answer "yes" when s/he really means "no" or "maybe." For example, "rather than refuse to the physician's face and cause him dishonor" (1991: 21), a Chinese woman described by Galanti told her physician that she would return for follow up treatment and then never did. Here is another example of this kind of situation.

ADELA SAMILLAN

Jackie, an Anglo nurse, was explaining the harmful side effects of the medication Adela Samillan, a Filipino patient, was to take at home after her discharge. Although Mrs. Samillan spoke some English, her husband, who was more fluent, served as interpreter. Throughout Jackie's explanation, the Samillans nodded in agreement and understanding and laughed nervously. When Jackie verbally tested them on the information, however, it was apparent that they understood very little. What had happened?

Dignity and self-esteem are extremely important for most Asians. Had the Samillans indicated that they did not understand Jackie's instructions, they would have lost their self-esteem for not understanding or they would have caused Jackie to lose hers for not explaining the material well enough. By pretending to understand, Mr. and Mrs. Samillan felt they were preserving everyone's dignity. (Galanti 1991: 20)

Shame

One of the quickest ways to injure client dignity is to write off their statements as old-fashioned or superstitious. A group of physicians interviewed by Robert Trotter told him that when a Mexican American mother said that her infant has *caída de mollera*, they "would tell the mother not to believe in that kind of 'superstitious nonsense' " (quoted in Arellano and Kearny 1992: 49). This was not an effective strategy.

Caída de mollera, or *mollera caída*, is a condition in which, among other things, an infant's anterior fontanel (the soft spot on the front of a baby's skull) is visibly depressed or has sunken or fallen in; the condition is also called "fallen fontanel." Other symptoms include excessive crying, reduced appetite, diarrhea, vomiting, restlessness, and irritability. The condition can be fatal without timely proper treatment; Trotter believes it is what biomedical specialists would call "severe dehydration." But because the women in Trotter's research knew that the clinicians would ridicule them, they would not bring the condition to the clinician's attention until it was very severe (Arellano and Kearny 1992: 49–50).

Clients' use of their own terms should not be denigrated but, rather, encouraged if clinicians are to provide adequate care; a client's use of the term caída de mollera can serve as a "good screening device" and a "significant indicator" that a child needs immediate attention (Arellano and Kearny 1992: 50). But how can clinicians find out about illnesses such as caída de mollera, let alone learn the terms for such illnesses, if clients are made to feel ashamed of them and then keep quiet?

The idea of becoming culturally sensitive may seem overwhelming in the face of all the possibilities. However, some common ethnographic methods can be incorporated into medical training and adapted and utilized by health care professionals to enhance relationships and care, as well as to complement medical science with medical art. Ultimately, even though mistakes will be made, they will be much less serious if there is an open, trusting, and mutually respectful relationship between practitioner and client.

ETHNOGRAPHIC TECHNIQUES: AN INTRODUCTION

Cultural sensitivity to communication practices, such as the ways in which the body is used or the people with whom it is appropriate to speak, is a first step in building sensitivity to other realms of culture. It is the first step in collecting and assessing further cultural data on a given aspect of a given way of life.

In order to enhance and facilitate communication, clinicians can try to gain an understanding of the beliefs, including those related to health, to which different client populations they serve subscribe—an ethnographic understanding. Technically, **ethnographies** are written accounts (-graphy) about certain peoples (ethno-). Libraries are full of such accounts, and this literature can be extremely helpful in familiarizing oneself with the culture of a client population.

In addition to library resources, original research can also be useful and rewarding. A growing number of clinicians are joining or forming study groups specifically interested in doing research on the populations they serve. There is also a growing number of resources and manuals directed to health care providers that summarize and give general information on techniques of rapid assessment (see Appendix, e.g., Fuller and Toon 1988; Kreps and Kunimoto 1994). H. Russell Bernard (1994) provides a full discussion of the methods professional ethnographers might use, as do Pelto and Pelto (1990).

The Ethnographic Assessment

While clinicians generally will not conduct full-fledged ethnographic research, they can collect ethnographic information by listening to what clients say about their lives. In order to gain insight into local social structures, clinicians should pay attention to the household forms most often described by clients. They also should attend to the types of individuals most often referred to by clients as emotional, social, and financial supports and those most often cited as barriers, trouble-makers, power brokers, or purse-string tighteners. Sometimes, in addition to individuals filling certain roles, such as that of father or cousin, specific community members occupying particular positions or offices will be named. The benevolence of those named community heroes may prove important if one wishes to gain the trust of the community.

One way clinicians can easily begin to collect social and cultural information is by getting out into the community and experiencing neighborhood life first hand. This can be done, for example, by eating lunch in a local park or restaurant rather than in the office. The interested clinician can ask a fellow worker or a long-time client who lives in or otherwise knows the area to accompany or guide her or him. Not only can this insider help to ease the clinician's entry, but his or her presence also might ensure the clinician's survival: some locations can be dangerous, especially in inner city areas.

Another way to increase awareness about the community being served is by paying attention to the media sources used by most members. Clinicians should find out what radio stations, newspapers, magazines, and TV shows or stations clinic clients listen to, read, and watch. Clinicians can ask clients directly; short discussions about the media may be good for increasing clients' comfort level in the service site as well as for assisting clinicians in building a community profile. Clinicians can use what they learn not only for their own erudition, but also to ensure that their waiting rooms are stocked with reading material that clients find pertinent. We are reminded of a participant in Sobo's AIDS research (1997) who remarked that the waiting room of the agency supposedly serving HIV-positive gay men had no gay newspapers or magazines. Unfortunately, this suggested to the man that he was not welcome there.

Participant Observation

The main ethnographic method traditionally has been **participant observation (PO)**, in which the fieldworker participates as fully as possible in the regular life of the community while observing all that goes on. Nonparticipant observation can also be done through simply observing and recording the observations without any notable participation in what is being observed.

Good PO demands good concentration, observation, and memory skills, all of which can be developed over time. For reasons discussed above, knowing how to communicate also is important; one who speaks the local language is more likely to learn about sensitive issues than those who do not (Naroll 1962, as cited in Bernard 1994: 145).

Key Informants

A clinician can also build a network of people traditionally called key informants. Key or "good informants are people to whom you can talk easily, who understand the information you need, and who are glad to give it to you or get it for you" (Bernard 1994: 166). Key informants generally have the ability to intellectualize their culture and, if apprised of the theories that the researcher is formulating, will be able to tell her or him if s/he is on the right track.

Key informants are strategically chosen; they are selected for their specialized knowledge. As Bernard notes, "In any given domain of culture, some people are more competent than others" (1994: 171). This makes the process of sampling, in which people are selected for their representativeness of the population in question, unnecessary for this kind of ethnographic inquiry.

For example, if one wished to find out about medicinal plants and their uses, the best person to ask would be an expert in that area. This would be much more efficient in terms of both time and effort than asking people randomly to tell you what they knew about that cultural domain.

Unstructured Data Collection

One gathers data from key informants and other informants or, rather, **participants**—people willing to help with and participate in the research but not so intensively—through ethnographic interviews. Single interviews can be helpful, but repeated interviews carried out over time with the same individuals generally generate more valid and reliable information as trust accrues.

PO entails constant **informal interviews**—casual, unplanned conversations in which important cultural facts are conveyed. For clinicians, however, much useful information can be collected through the clinical interview or consultation.

While informal interviews are "characterized by a total lack of structure or control," **formal interviews**, like clinical interviews, involve purposefully sitting down with an informant to talk about a given topic (Bernard 1994: 209). Formal interviews can be unstructured or structured. As Bernard shows, "there is a continuum of interview situations based on the amount of control we try to exercise over the responses of informants" (209).

The **unstructured interview** would generally be the type conducted during the early stages of clinical contact as a way of simply warming people up to the idea of your interest in their culture and as a way of determining what kinds of questions structured interviews should entail. H. Russell Bernard, whose work forms the basis of much of our methods discussion, suggests, "Tell everyone you interview that you are trying to learn from *them*. Encourage them to interrupt you during the interview with anything they think is important" (1994: 211; emphasis in original). Let client or participant concerns guide the flow of discussion. The ethnographer-clinician's greatest skill is to listen—a skill that should already be a part of the clinician's role and repertoire.

The emergent concerns of the participant should override predetermined questions at any time if the questions prove to be irrelevant, misguided, or culturally biased. A culturally biased question is one that forces a participant to think about an issue that s/he would not otherwise consider. People generally can come up with an answer, but if that answer never comes into play in real-life, it is of little use to the clinician. Patients that are asked culturally biased questions also often tend to respond with what they think the practitioner wants to hear (cf. Bernard 1994: 231).

Culturally biased questions include those in which the categories used are those of the interviewer, not the interviewee. For example, Sobo has demonstrated (1996a) how abortion, as defined from a biomedical (etic) standpoint, may not be perceived as such by those being queried; Jamaicans, for example, like many other peoples, do not consider extracting a late menstrual period (menstrual regulation) as abortion. There are many reasons for this, one being that a fetus is not seen as a humanized potential baby until it becomes active in the womb, which generally happens about four or five months after conception.

This example demonstrates how essential it is to find out how informants define terms or categories from their point of view before naively using categories in assessments. In the unstructured interview, a number of probing techniques are used to elicit such emic information. These include the

silent probe, which Bernard defines as "just remaining quiet and waiting for an informant to continue" (215), sometimes with a nod or a mumbled "uh-huh." A positive probe involves an overtly stated "yes" or "I see." An **echo probe** encourages a participant to continue by echoing the last word or phrase that s/he said, in a questioning tone. ("Questioning tone?") Yes, the questioning tone provokes further elaboration. Another way to do so is to construct a probe such that extensive information is needed to respond to it, such as, "Tell me all the things you might do to stop diarrhea in your baby."

One also might use information to get information, as in suggesting that you already know why parents feed their children milk when you really do not know this at all. *If you have built up good relationships with your interviewees*, they will correct you when you are wrong or confirm your hypothesis and fill you in on the details you were missing. Further, in regard to sensitive topics, by appearing to know more than you do know, participants can be made to feel that "*they* are not the ones who are giving away the 'secrets' of the group, or that they are not actually divulging anything" (Bernard 1994: 219; emphasis in original). However, because of the ethical dilemma that the latter use of this technique can entail, it should only be used in a carefully considered fashion.

Structured Data Collection

One of the main points of ethnography is to collect data concerning the issues as participants see them. This can be done with structured, as well as unstructured, methods. **Structured** data collection methods are used "to control the input that triggers each informant's responses so that the output can be reliably compared" (Bernard 1994: 237). Questionnaires, for example, fit this bill.

Using a questionnaire is a way of conducting survey research, or research in which a large number of people, generally a carefully selected sample, are polled. **Questionnaires** generally consist of a page or several pages of questions that participants are asked to answer. Questionnaires can be administered in person, by mail, over the phone, or in a variety of other ways. For clinicians, brief questionnaires might be included with the required paperwork patients fill out on arriving for appointments.

The questions on questionnaires can be closed or open-ended. **Closed**, or forced choice, questions force the participant to choose between two or more options. Sometimes the answers are provided in scale form (e.g., never, rarely, sometimes, often, always). **Open-ended** questions are those for which respondents can answer as they like. The major themes that emerge in these answers can be identified and a coding scheme generated so that, as with closed-answer questionnaires, data collected can be quantified for processing.

One of the main problems in questionnaire construction is ambiguity, so that each respondent answers what is, in the end, a different set of questions, making the results less useful than they might be. This has been made clear in HIV and AIDS research where, for example, the phrase "sexually active" can have many meanings. Precision is key, and often this means conducting unstructured research before constructing a questionnaire so that you can be sure of the meanings that respondents will attribute to the words used in the questions—and to be sure that your answer options, and your questions themselves, are not perceived as ridiculous.

Questions and Answers

"The multicultural person," notes Hoopes, "is the person who has learned how to learn culture—rapidly and effectively" (1981: 10–38). Health care providers must strive to become multicultural individuals— "individuals who have mastered the knowledge and skills necessary to feel comfortable and communicate effectively with people of similar and dissimilar backgrounds, in any situation involving a group of people of diverse ethnocultural backgrounds" (Majumdar 1995: chapter 4, 2).

In becoming more multicultural, clinicians can benefit by studying the work of others, by asking considered questions in the clinic, by taking the time to learn how to ask these questions so that they make sense to the client, by actually listening to the answers, and by otherwise familiarizing themselves with the cultural and social milieu in which clients live. Awareness, coupled with the proper skills for cultural assessment (Majumdar 1995), can allow for identifying the variables appropriate to specific cases and client populations, and provide a more personal and empathetic understanding not only of one's clients, but of oneself. Helpful references for further skill development and cultural sensitivity training are included in the Appendix.

It is not our intention to provide a catalog of ethnic practices or a crosscultural file in which health care workers can look up the patterned health practices of particular peoples. That approach not only leads to stereotyping, but decontextualizes human interaction and goes against the holism entailed in the culture concept. Rather, then, the examples are meant to alert the reader to areas in which differences might be located and to the cultural processes or cultural logics that can underlie actions. This kind of alertness helps the practitioner assess individual clients with respect to various culturally based behaviors and motivations.

Our goal is to encourage cultural sensitivity, or an awareness that one group's habitual actions and patterns of thought cannot be assumed to be the same as those of people from other societies or cultures. Moreover, they should not be noticed only when pathological or identified solely as such. As Locke notes,

Multicultural efforts must focus on normal behaviors and wellness, rather than on abnormal behaviors and illness. Far too many efforts at meeting the needs of ethnically diverse individuals fail because they begin from a viewpoint of abnormality rather than normality. Factors such as "low self-esteem" and "self-hatred" are frequently assumed to be characteristic of ethnically diverse group members without any investigation of the basis on which such claims are made. We must also use care in how we translate research results and generalize them to populations larger than those used in the research investigations. (Locke 1992: 160)

Ileana Herrell of the U.S. Public Health Office of Minority Health also gives cautionary advice. As she points out, there is a growing number of highly individual racial and ethnic groups, and we are only "slowly learning just what tools will work in diagnosing and treating their health care needs" (1992: 8). Herrell states that information is only beginning to reach the public health and health care mainstream as to just how different groups may be in their health beliefs, practices, and needs, and that data is outdated almost as soon as it is received. This implies urgent need for behavioral research (11).

Beliefs and practices related to ethnicity, although a major focus of multiculturalism, are not the only variables important to health. Herrell stresses the interconnections of ethnicity, socioeconomic status, age, and gender. It is, after all, an individual who is being treated. The benefits of taking time to appreciate the emic, or insider's, point of view are very apparent in relation to HIV and AIDS, as well as in any integration of modalities and expansion of the model of medical care, which the following chapter examines.

QUESTIONS FOR DISCUSSION

1. If you were caring for a patient whose language you did not speak, what would you do? What qualities would you look for in a translator to ensure full and forthright communication?

2. What are some of the nonverbal forms of communication that health care workers should be sensitive to? How might their meanings, significances, and subtleties vary cross-culturally?

3. If you took a job in a clinic far from your home that served a cultural group with which you were unfamiliar, how might you go about collecting information that would enhance your practice, enabling you to offer culturally sensitive care to your clients?

4. What are the benefits of unstructured, as opposed to structured, data collection? What are the various techniques of unstructured data collection?

7

Application and Integration: Contemporary Challenges

Change is inevitable, and it is the hope of men and women of good will that change will be for the better—better for society and for each individual. Voluntary reform is a saner and healthier form of change than explosive measures taken as a result of abuse. It is time for analysis and reform in our medical schools and in the medical centers where interns and residents are trained if medicine—as both a science and an art—is to meet the needs of our time. Even the most thoughtful and probing analysis will be imperfect. Even the most earnestly pursued remedies will not be wholly successful. But if we cannot reach the ideal, we can move toward it. At the very least we will have had the sense and courage to try.

[Cook 1972: 211]

Goal: To be able to draw constructively on the various concepts discussed in previous chapters in an integrative fashion to understand how we might better cope with specific diseases, like HIV/AIDS, and to be able to generate ideas for future action.

Goal: To gain an understanding, from concrete examples, of how health program policy makers and practitioners can productively bring cultural and social factors to bear on health issues, and how sociocultural medicine can be actualized.

Robin Cook, M.D., wrote those words on reform in 1972. It is arguable whether we have moved closer to the ideal or whether we, as a nation, even know what it is. What is apparent is that our problems and our future solutions are inextricably linked to our social and cultural context, with all its difficulties, richness, and diversity.

For all of us, our social structures will determine, to a large extent, our life chances, risks, barriers, and opportunities. We all hope to be healthy or physically and mentally able to pursue whatever we feel is worth pursuing, and we hope to be supported in our pursuits by others who care about us.

We have much in common as human beings who enter and leave this world in essentially the same way. We all die, whatever that death may mean to us and to those we love; we also develop various options for response when we become ill. Although we all face many difficulties in dealing with problems of illness, disability, and death, the diversity of our cultures and our approaches to problems testifies to human resilience and imagination.

This chapter first ties together previously presented concepts by focusing on a specific health problem: **AIDS, or Acquired Immune Deficiency Syndrome**. It demonstrates the role of social structure, cultural norms, and values, exploring the limitations to recognition and care in the disease's spread, and suggests a much broader approach to meeting vital needs that are not addressed by the biomedical model. This chapter then examines the possibility of integrating biomedical with nonbiomedical approaches across the board so that our health system can more adequately meet the challenges of the future.

AIDS: AN OVERVIEW

Today, the cumulative number of reported AIDS cases in the United States is over half a million. More than 60 percent of these people have already died. AIDS is the leading cause of death among American men aged 25 to 44; it is the third leading cause for women in this age range (CDC 1995: 5).

Most of the people now suffering from AIDS were infected years ago with **Human Immunodeficiency Virus (HIV)**, the virus that breaks down the human immune system, making the infected individual vulnerable to AIDS. According to CDC estimates, perhaps 75 million U.S. residents, or about one in three hundred, are infected with HIV (McQuillan et al. 1994), although infection is not evenly distributed throughout the population.

HIV-positive, or HIV-infected, U.S. residents account for only about 5 percent of the 15 million individuals worldwide infected with HIV. U.S. AIDS cases represent only about 10 percent of the 3 million people worldwide who have AIDS or have died from it (WHO 1994). This chapter describes the **pandemic** (worldwide epidemic) that has caused so much death and suffering, and it shows how culture influences both risks for and responses to AIDS.

The word epidemic refers both to the rapid spread of a disease and to a disease that is prevalent in a given locality. But as AIDS has covered the globe so thoroughly, pandemic is a more applicable term. In addition, as Robert Searles Walker points out, AIDS is not a plague.

Plague is a theological idea; it refers to an event that is imputed to God. In our emotional memory, plagues are terrifying, devastating, inescapable expressions of God's wrath and judgment. Those who die in them are targets. . . . Epidemics, no matter how serious, pale into insignificance before direct manifestations of divine anger. The word "epidemic" is a term associated with the science of public health. Epidemics are understandable aspects of nature and manageable with modern skills. People who die in them are unfortunate victims, not sinners. Epidemics come from a nonjudgmental "Nature". . . . Plagues come from God. (Walker 1991: 3)

Recall our discussion of magic in chapter 4. As Walker writes, "Words can heal; words can kill. In the AIDS epidemic, 'plague' is a lethal, killer word. The mindset expressed by the word excused the slowness and weakness of governmental action at the national, state, and local levels" (1991: 4).

Ground Zero

In 1989, Job Bwayo opened a free clinic for the truckers near Nairobi, Kenya. Blood tests revealed that 27 percent of them were HIV-positive (Conover 1993: 57). That is, more than one in four had HIV antibodies in their blood, indicating that HIV was also present. Dr. Bwayo was not surprised and may have even been relieved that things were not worse.

AIDS is **endemic** (locally prevalent, a common problem) in this section of Africa. In Uganda, the seropositivity rate in the early 1990s was 36 percent; in Rwanda, it was 51 percent (Conover 1993: 57). That we have these statistics at all is fortunate. African AIDS resources are extremely limited. By the time most individuals are diagnosed as being sick from AIDS, they are usually close to death.

Modernization and the Spread of AIDS

AIDS's bodily effects are staggering, especially when we consider HIV's fragility. HIV easily dies once out of the body, and it cannot go anywhere without a human host to transport it. Our bodies are the virus's chauffeurs. Were it not for certain social structural changes spurred by global capitalist interests in Africa, including the **demographic** changes (population shifts) brought about by modernization, HIV would probably still be living an isolated country life in a remote part of central Africa, where it seems to have originated more than forty years ago.

The growth of transcontinental trade and trucking; the rise in automobile, bus, and train travel; and the related increase in urbanization, and therefore of urban migration, enabled HIV's spread. As we moved from village to city—and from nation to nation—we carried the virus with us much as we carried our baggage.

Migration to cities by those seeking work and the growth of the capitalistic cash economy—which has historically denied women fair wages—led to a rise in urban prostitution, as urban men sought sex from urban women who found themselves in need of money. High rates of untreated sexually transmitted diseases (STDs) among impoverished people, and the open genital ulcers that untreated STDs usually entail, increase the likelihood for infection by giving HIV instant access to the body. When infected urban migrants return to their villages for visits, they carry HIV back into the countryside. The rapid increase of intercontinental jet travel and the movement of medical and religious missions, government representatives, business people, and especially soldiers and tourists from one part of the globe to another gave the virus an even broader range of motion.

Condoms

While latex condoms have been available for years in many parts of Africa, there as elsewhere they often are not used. This is partly because of the high cultural value placed on children. But it also has to do with more immediate cost-benefit calculations. For example, in one establishment frequented by African truckers, condoms cost 200 shillings apiece. When a room for the night costs 400 shillings, a prostitute 400–600, a meal 100, and when there are dependent kin at home, 200 shillings will seem a lot to spend on a little bit of latex (Conover 1993: 60).

Truckers interviewed by Ted Conover introduced him to an innkeeper named Bora at one of their stops, and among the news she had for them as they relaxed in the pub was a story about a man who had recently died of AIDS: "It turned out that when the authorities went to the house . . . they found dozens of packages of unused condoms [with] dates that had expired! Knowing murmurs circled the table, and I asked Francis [a trucker] to explain. 'These condoms, when they are too old, contain germs,' he said. 'And that's how he got AIDS' " (1993: 68).

Poor-quality condoms are not unique to Africa. And their quality probably did not start out as poor. But hot weather and shipping delays can lead to latex deterioration. Problems also can result because clinicians fail to or do not have time to provide clients with full instructions on how condoms are to be cared for, used, and taken off.

Other modernization-related hazards that foster the spread of AIDS include increased civil strife and warfare over territory and resources that lead to blood baths and violent rape, which increase exposure to HIV.

Spread of technology has also increased use of injections and reuse of contaminated needles and other equipment that is in short supply in economically poorer nations. In addition, there is simply not enough money to test the safety of blood supplies available for transfusions, which may also transmit HIV. Clearly, effectively combating AIDS means combating a whole range of problems raised by the modernization processes and by the unequal distribution of wealth and health within and between nations that modernization entails.

AIDS in the World

Nearly 70 percent of the world's HIV-positive individuals live in Africa. Masses of orphans have been created. About one-third of all children borne by infected women will have AIDS themselves. Kin networks that would ordinarily care for the orphans and the sick children may be structurally too weak to do so because so many family members have died off. Once-productive villages are no longer self-sufficient; labor shortages can lead to famine, increasing vulnerability to HIV infection.

Some estimate that by the year 2000, East Asia will emerge as the region with the greatest proportion of HIV-positive individuals (Kammerer and Symonds 1992). The growing prominence of AIDS in East Asia and the key role of heterosexual transmission is linked to the massive, pervasive (mostly heterosexual) sex trade.

While AIDS is spread worldwide mostly through heterosexual intercourse, in the United States and in Europe, HIV found its first stronghold in the homosexual male population. Bisexuality in men has become a major factor in transmitting HIV to women, as women may have heterosexual intercourse with bisexual men. Bisexuality in men may be more common where homosexuality is not condoned, as men will then supplement overt heterosexual relations with covert homosexual ones (see also chapter 2).

Religion, which like bisexuality is, in some cases, linked with homophobia, also plays a part in the AIDS pandemic. Condom use may be forbidden, as it is by the Catholic church. Catholicism also idealizes virginity, and this can, in some contexts, lead girls and women to engage in anal sex. Catholicism is strong in certain Hispanic or Latino communities. Young Latina women comprise one of the fastest growing groups of people living with HIV or AIDS (PWHAs) in the United States.

WHAT EXACTLY IS AIDS? DEFINITION DEBATES

AIDS, or Acquired Immune Deficiency Syndrome, is an end result of infection with HIV, or Human Immunodeficiency Virus. We create HIV antibodies, and the presence of these are what HIV tests measure. This immune response notwithstanding, HIV invades and destroys our T-cells, white blood cells that are essential to the proper functioning of the immune system. AIDS is the label applied to those whose immune systems have been severely challenged by HIV. As the immune system breaks down, one becomes exceptionally susceptible to disease; even a common cold can kill.

Infections that set in as the immune system begins to fail and AIDS materializes are called **opportunistic infections**. Progression from HIV infection to AIDS is determined by whether or not a person has contracted certain of these infections or by a T-cell count of below 200. It is sometimes accompanied by massive weight loss.

The Centers for Disease Control and Prevention (CDC) maintains a list of **indicator diseases**—diseases that indicate the onset of AIDS. Certain diseases are considered key, and infection with just one of these is enough to qualify an individual as having AIDS.

As AIDS was first identified as such in homosexual men, the indicator disease list originally contained only the diseases diagnosed in these men. But AIDS in women reveals itself in different diseases. Because of this, and because clinicians often did not think to offer women HIV tests, many women with AIDS went undiagnosed.

Eventually, the CDC amended the indicator disease list to include opportunistic infections likely to strike women, such as invasive cervical cancer. After January 1, 1993, when the changes went into effect, the number of women diagnosed as having AIDS increased dramatically (CDC 1993a: 3).

The opportunistic infections that trouble HIV-infected individuals, male or female, include those caused by numerous viruses, fungi, bacteria, and protozoa. The microbes that attack the HIV-infested body are generally common, and they are normally easily disposed of by the immune system. But HIV infection disarms the immune system so that these microbes can proliferate freely, leading to frequent and severe bouts with disease. As an HIV-positive woman commenting on the ironic nature of rejection and fear of HIV-positive people on the part of the general public said: "Some people just totally freak, and [say] 'Oh my god she's HIV positive!' and 'She has AIDS!' And they're coughing all over me and gossiping at the same time. And I'm thinking, 'Don't you know that cold can kill me?'" (Sobo 1995).

TESTING POSITIVE

Getting Tested

The ramifications of a positive diagnosis with HIV or AIDS can be enormous. Those who get tested—and return for their results—often find the lexicon or vocabulary that clinicians use confusing, and this can lead to mistaken interpretations of results. For instance, tested individuals sometimes understand positive results as "good" or as indicating that one is free of HIV, when the opposite is the case. Further, people who think that they have "passed" the HIV test sometimes equate their perceived negative status with immunity, and this can lead to an attitude of carelessness or even to an increase in risk behavior (Kurth and Hutchison 1989). Those involved in testing and counseling should concentrate on clearly conveying meanings by translating medical jargon into plain English (or other appropriate languages), and they should double-check clients' understandings to make sure that they are correct.

Positive Results

If test results are **positive**, the testee must adjust to his or her new status as a **PWHA (person living with HIV or AIDS)**. The individual's psychological reaction is influenced by his or her own cultural beliefs and the perceived cultural beliefs of members of his or her social networks.

Individual identity constructions affect how people deal with HIV seropositivity. William Borden found that "HIV seropositivity is likely to threaten existing interpretations of self, others, life experience, and anticipated future" (1991: 438). In other words, a positive HIV test may entail a need to revise one's life history, and this can be devastating. In some cases, one must adjust to fears about infecting partners and children or about abandoning them through death. Coping with HIV or AIDS also involves grieving for and ultimately accepting the loss of one's future as well as accepting the uncertainty that comes with new diseases such as this.

AIDS carries a culturally constructed **stigma** or mark of disgrace that most other chronic diseases do not, and this often leads to intense social and moral confusion for the infected individual. Some may feel unable to inform friends and family, which can lead to "increased isolation during a time of great need" (Kurth and Hutchison 1989: 262). Partners may not be told, for fear that they might become violent or will end the relationship.

To Tell or Not to Tell?

In light of the foregoing, it will be clear that, while to many seronegative people self-disclosure seems an imperative and obvious step, the seropositive weigh a number of factors to determine whether or not and to whom they will disclose their status. These factors are intimately linked with cultural assumptions about HIV and AIDS.

Because self-disclosure is so potentially dangerous, deciding when and if to do it is a complex matter. In a study of self-disclosure of a number of conditions deemed stigmatizing in the United States, including HIV seropositivity, Limandri (1989) found that the disclosee's responses to the information disclosed and to the self-discloser himself or herself are key.

Generally, the self-discloser will "conceal for awhile, disclose, then retract back into concealment" (73), searching for some sign that his or her full revelation will not result in rejection.

Findings from a U.S. study concerning self-disclosure show that the main reasons for nondisclosure included (1) not wanting to worry or upset others, (2) fear of discrimination, (3) fear of disrupting relationships, (4) emotional self-protection, (5) feeling that the person told would have little beneficial to offer, (6) a lack of closeness with the individual, and (7) the desire to conceal one's homosexuality (Hays et al. 1993). Importantly, many of the men who participated in this study said that they planned to tell most people, but "the timing was not yet right" (1993: 430).

RISK GROUPS

Despite intergroup differences, high-risk behavior cuts across ethnic, class, sexual identity, and other so-called boundaries. Still, certain groups seem more prone to contract AIDS than others. It is tempting to single out particular groups as risk groups—as bounded groups that, by virtue of some essential traits particular to the members of each, are at a high risk for AIDS. But one's risk for infection has more to do with geography and history than with ethnic, national, sexual, or other aspects of one's identity. So, while aspects of identity may serve as **risk markers**, they are not in themselves **risk factors**. In the following sections, we identify some of the behavioral, socioeconomic, and historical risk factors that make certain groups more vulnerable to HIV and AIDS.

WOMEN AND AIDS

The underreporting of AIDS in women notwithstanding, women account for half of all AIDS cases in much of sub-Saharan Africa and in parts of the Caribbean. Women worldwide are currently being infected three times as quickly as men (*AIDS Alert* 1993). And most women get AIDS from men: heterosexual or male-to-female transmission accounts for 90 percent of all female cases of AIDS worldwide (*AIDS Alert* 1993), and for 37 percent of U.S. female cases (CDC 1995). In the United States, heterosexual transmission edged out intravenous drug use as the most common mode of female infection in 1992 (*JAMA* 1993). Importantly, heterosexual transmission does not just mean transmission that occurs during vaginal intercourse. Many heterosexuals have anal sex. At least 10 percent of American women aged 15 to 64 "engage with some frequency in anal intercourse," and 39 percent of American women have had at least one experience of anal sex (Voeller 1990).

Women are sociologically and biologically more vulnerable to heterosexual HIV infection than men are. Women involved in heterosexual intercourse are generally on the receptive or receiving end, which entails a biologically higher risk for infection than penetrative partners' experience does. When force is used, HIV-welcoming tissue damage is even more likely. Oral contraceptive use, the use of intrauterine contraceptive devices, and vaginal or other reproductive tract infections increase women's susceptibility to HIV (Bezemer 1992).

Worldwide, 70 percent of all new female infectees are between the ages of 15 and 25 (Rensberger 1993). The younger a woman is, the thinner her vaginal lining is, making her more biologically vulnerable than older women. And young women are sociologically vulnerable: they often have sex with men who are older than they and have, therefore, had more opportunity for acquiring an HIV infection. Further, young women often have anal sex as a way of protecting their (vaginal) virginity.

It is probably not the one-night stand who transfers HIV to women: most are infected by steady male partners. But multiple partnering may increase a woman's risk for other sexually transmitted diseases, thereby making her more vulnerable to HIV infection during sex with her primary partner (Nichols 1990; see also Reiss 1991, as cited in Bolton 1992).

The quality of gender relations and the structure of gender-linked power differentials also affect women's risk for infections. According to one study, men are significantly more likely than women to have lied in the negotiation of safer sex (35 percent versus 10 percent; Cochran 1989).

AIDS AND WOMEN OF COLOR IN THE UNITED STATES

Gender-linked risk factors will differ across groups. Three-quarters (74.6 percent) of female AIDS cases in the United States are members of minority groups. Black women are about fourteen times more likely than white women to be diagnosed with AIDS (Campbell 1990). The situation for other women of color, such as Latinas, is similarly grim.

The forces leading to unsafe sexual practice are found universally, to greater or lesser degrees, in different sociocultural contexts. Rates of certain kinds of high-risk practices are lower among black women than among Whites (e.g., Lewis and Watters 1989; Weinberg and Williams 1988; see also Wilson 1987; Worth 1990). But despite the fact that, overall, black women seem to take fewer sexual risks than white women, black women's AIDS rates are higher. Urban poverty plays a huge role here.

As in impoverished nations, the conditions of life in the inner-city make unsafe sex among those who live there particularly likely to lead to HIV infection. Economic oppression (and the effects of this on gender relations), substandard health care, the frequency of injectable drug use, high rates of untreated STDs, and other typical inner-city and poverty-related conditions exacerbate the effects that unsafe sex practices have on the rate of HIV transmission among urban Blacks. Upon diagnosis, the average remaining life expectancy for Whites is between eighteen and twenty-four months. For Blacks, it is only six months (Lester and Saxxon 1988).

There are also cultural reasons for the disparities in HIV transmission rates. Among Blacks as among most peoples, cultural norms for sexuality differ between men and women. Men are expected to have active extra-conjugal sex lives, while women are not. This is generally traced to man's lack of economic opportunity and his related dependence on favorable peer evaluations (Anderson 1990; Liebow 1967). William Oliver (1989) explains the "complex of values and norms that characterize the way many lower-class Black males define manhood"—a complex that includes "the tough guy and the player-of-women images"—as a "cultural adaptation to white racism" and a "compensatory adaptation" (260, 261). Following Hannerz, Oliver calls this complex "compulsive masculinity" (Hannerz 1969, as cited in Oliver: 261).

In a world where male homicide, incarceration, underemployment, and unemployment rates run high, "good" men are hard to find. Many women therefore ignore men's infidelity as men share their time and (sometimes) their money with a number of partners. This limits the social, emotional, and (sometimes) financial resources that each partner receives.

Men are often eager to sire offspring as proof of their heterosexual activity, and women can have children to please and bind men—to establish kinship-type links with them and their kin (M. Ward 1990). Childbearing also can be a way of trying to improve one's status: each child born holds the promise of achieving great things and of reflecting well on the mother, as well as of being a source of joy and unconditional love. Knowing that the supply of marriageable or employed men is very small, some women choose to build families and network connections without the perceived burden of a husband or boyfriend. But unprotected sex, necessary in many cases for male support (whether social, emotional, or financial) and always needed for conception, entails HIV and STD risks.

OPTIMISM AND RISK (MIS)PERCEPTION

As Fischoff and colleagues argue, the "choice of an option depends upon all of its features, not just its risk" (1981: 134). The risk of HIV infection, and therefore of AIDS, is just one of many risks faced daily by impoverished urban minority women. Under such conditions, the benefits of heterosexual interaction and of possible pregnancy and childbearing outweigh the risk of disease, when not risking disease could lead to more immediate consequences such as verbal or physical abuse, the loss of a partner, or childlessness. All of these consequences involve concrete hardship as well as lowered status and damaged self-esteem.

Relevant cultural knowledge and information about culture-specific role expectations are essential for developing predictions of when and how specific kinds of AIDS risk denial will occur and strategies to combat this denial and so to reduce risk behaviors and control the spread of AIDS. No matter what one's objective risk level is, in the context of mainstream American culture believing or indicating that one is at risk for AIDS would involve admitting one's failure to live up to standards for prudent sexual (or drug-related) behavior (the shortcomings of these standards notwithstanding). Because such an admission could have dire effects on self-esteem, identity, and status, many people maintain what Neil Weinstein (1989) has called **optimistically biased** AIDS risk denial. That is, they play down or ignore their own risks for HIV infection; they fail to apply to themselves or to personalize messages regarding AIDS risks.

Frightening thoughts of one's susceptibility, social marginality, and impending physical and, moreover, social death need not be confronted if one's AIDS risk is denied. Further, denial allows a person to preserve her own self-esteem and status, just as admitting to the risk by using condoms can lower self-esteem. This is because denying one's risk for AIDS involves denying that one engages in stigmatized practices, including what are perceived as unwise partnering choices.

By denying risk, people can not only preserve but also raise their status and self-esteem, as denying one's own risk implicitly—and sometimes explicitly—involves asserting that others are at a higher risk for the problem than oneself. Indeed, people often report that their peers' risk levels for negative outcomes like AIDS are higher than their own. In part, this is because people tend to compare themselves to stereotypic images of those who take few or no self-protective actions; that is, we compare ourselves to high-risk individuals rather than to our actual peers (Weinstein 1989: 1982).

Katherine Kinsey (1994) conducted a study of the HIV- and AIDS-related knowledge, attitudes, and beliefs of about 100 urban women, most of whom were members of minority groups. Kinsey observed participants' use of what she called distancing maneuvers to maintain denial. For example, one of the participants optimistically stated: "I know four brothers (all drug abusers) who have AIDS but I don't do what they do and besides they live in a different neighborhood" (83). Participants also misused negative HIV test results to support their self-affirming contentions that they were not at risk for contracting the virus.

The cognitive or thought process of optimistic bias seems to have no link with a person's actual risk level (Hansen, Hahn, and Wolkenstein 1990; Weinstein 1989). Landesman and colleagues (1987, in Nichols 1990) interviewed 602 poor, urban, nonwhite new mothers in New York; the women also were tested for HIV antibodies. Two-thirds of the women who tested positive did not know that they were at risk. Similar findings were reported by a team of researchers (Lindsay et al. 1989) in Atlanta who conducted HIV tests for 3,472 inner-city minority women during pregnancy. "If we had followed [recommendations only to test women with self-reported risk factors]," the researchers said, "more than 70% of our seropositive women would not have been identified, because they did not self-acknowledge risk factors" (293).

Although not linked to actual risk levels, optimistic bias does have a strong tie to the degree to which a condition is stigmatized (Prohaska, Albrecht, and Levy 1990). It also has a strong tie to a risk's perceived preventability (Weinstein 1989). As Weinstein writes, "The more preventable the hazard, the greater the threat to self-esteem" (1989: 157), and the greater the threat to self-esteem, the more useful optimistic bias can be. This makes the job of the AIDS prevention counselor in the United States even more difficult, as AIDS is seen as preventable by many Americans.

AIDS TREATMENTS

Seeking Healing

What medical experiences await the seropositive? In the developing world, biomedical care for PWHAs is scarce. Even so, PWHAs there do procure medical treatment of many kinds. Among Haitians, for example, treatment often consists of prayer and perhaps a few pain killers. AIDS is not always seen as a simple communicable disease: in certain cases, it is explained as having been sent by God or through sorcery by an enemy. So, sometimes people consult Voodoo, or Vodoun, priests.

Vodoun is Haiti's traditional indigenous religion. A hybrid of African and Catholic traditions, Vodoun, like any religion, provides explanations for misfortune, and its rituals have healing power. Many people of Haitian as well as other Caribbean origins living in the United States practice diffused and adapted versions of this religion.

If AIDS has been sent as a hex or curse, sometimes the priest works to send misfortune back to the person who arranged to send it to begin with. He or she also works to cure the PWHA. Often, this entails holding public ceremonies to please the spirit world. Such ceremonies generally consist of much drumming, dancing, singing, and praying, and food is offered to the gods. Participants often are possessed by spirits enticed to visit by the congregation's festivities. Priests also work private rituals for the sick. Sometimes, they mix medicines from herbs and other ingredients.

The Haitian example demonstrates that people will use their traditional health beliefs to explain and manage, or try to manage, modern health threats. George Rivera Jr.'s work concerning responses to AIDS among Mexican Americans and Mexicans living near the U.S.–Mexico border provides another example of this (1990). Many Mexicans and Mexican Americans subscribe to the healing system called *Curanderismo*, in which indigenous healers known as *curanderos* (male) or *curanderas* (female) are consulted. Like Vodoun, Curanderismo provides explanations and treatments for numerous health problems. These include plant-based medicines, prayer, or magical rites, such as the burning of candles.

Rivera interviewed a number of curandero/as and found that while some felt that they could not treat AIDS, others had devised treatment plans modeled on traditional treatments for illnesses involving symptoms similar to those exhibited with AIDS. However, they did not see AIDS as related to these illnesses. And they did not explain AIDS as the result of witchcraft or sorcery. Instead, the healers considered AIDS as a new communicable disease brought on by excess pollution in the body, an imbalance of acids, or the body's invasion by *mal aire*, or evil (bad, tainted) air. Those who thought it incurable recommended praying to St. Lazarus, who was raised from the dead, as they would for people with any incurable illness.

People the world over pick and choose from all available systems—traditional and modern, folk and professional—when devising their therapy regimens. PWHAs living in San Francisco, California, might combine biomedical attention with Chinese herbalism; PWHAs living in Santa Fe, New Mexico, might add Curanderismo and New Age crystal therapy to their biomedical treatment regimes. One in four people using biomedical means to treat a health problem also are using other modalities (Eisenberg et al. 1993; see also chapter 4).

Delivery of Care by the U.S. Public Health System

The experiences of poor black women demonstrate the social, economic, and cultural dimensions of health care in the U.S. public health system. As Martha Ward observes, "The diagnosis of HIV only adds another bureaucracy and another layer of complications to an already burdened life" (1993b: 59). HIV seropositivity is not generally an inner-city woman's worst problem: as Ward found, there are often other sick people in the family, as well as children to feed and rent to be paid. Because of gender expectations, like most mainstream women, urban women with HIV or AIDS often feel that they must take care of others before they take care of themselves. They frequently find it easier to bring a sick child to the doctor than to go in for their own appointments (and while some clinics have recently tried group appointments for the convenience of their clients, adults and children often must go to different clinics, on different days). Clinicians are often more sympathetic toward pediatric AIDS cases than they are toward sick women. "In New Orleans," writes Ward, "we have cases where many service providers, professionals, and volunteers attend the funeral of a baby dead from AIDS; not one of them is present at the mother's funeral" (1993b: 60).

Many women learn that they are seropositive only after being tested in the course of prenatal care. If there is time, pressure is often put on them to undergo an abortion.

All babies carry maternal antibodies, and so all babies born to HIV-infected women carry their mothers' antibodies for HIV. But in nearly two out of three cases, these antibodies disappear after about sixteen months (as do other maternal antibodies). An infected woman's chances of giving birth to a healthy child, then, are relatively high: less than one-third of all babies born to HIV-positive mothers will develop AIDS. In light of the other odds and obstacles that inner-city women face daily, and in light of the joy that a child can bring, this gamble can seem minimal. Besides, current legal restrictions, social and cultural pressures, financial problems, and clinicians' misgivings about exposing themselves to HIV make getting an abortion very difficult for seropositive inner-city women who would chose to do so.

While losing a wanted child is bad enough, abortion can lead to other social losses. Partners, friends, and family members who know of one's pregnancy may demand an explanation; revealing one's seropositivity may result in abandonment. For some black Americans, social losses go beyond one's immediate relations: abortion is, in some people's minds, a tool for genocide (the planned elimination of a specific cultural or ethnic group). As Levine and Dubler write, "Efforts to stem the spread of HIV through the control of reproduction may be seen as attempts to destroy the African-American and Latino communities" (1990: 334).

Pregnant or not, quality health care often is beyond the reach of inner-city women infected with HIV. In addition to health care that often is not covered by what little insurance an inner-city woman has (assuming she has any), an ill woman must find a way to pay for transportation to appointments, child care, and so forth. Drugs for HIV-related conditions can be prohibitively expensive. Further, many have not been tested on women, whose susceptibility to HIV infection was ignored until recently.

Besides their problems linked to class and gender, PWHAs of color suffer from racism in the health care system. It is manifested in cursory physical examinations, inadequate bed assignments, delayed admissions, and assumptions of noncompliance. Racism often overlaps with discrimination against the poor, and it influences the adoption, implementation, and administration of health policies that negatively affect the lives of lower-income people (Hutchinson 1993).

Confidentiality or secrecy is also a major issue for most infected women. For caregivers, clients' desires to control knowledge of their infections poses logistical headaches (how to remember who has and who has not been informed of each client's status?) and ethical ones, especially when clients are minors or when their children have AIDS. Further, their confidentiality concerns lead these women to shy away from using the services of supportive community organizations, which they view with suspicion and see as intrusive and scrutinizing.

Mays and Cochran point out that impoverished black HIV-positive women may emphasize secrecy more than other seropositive people do because "the impact of rejection for Blacks may be more severe, given existing cultural norms emphasizing the kinship network as the provider of both tangible and emotional social support" (1987: 227). Infected women who also are mothers may feel their kin will be more likely to care for their children after they die if the cause of death is kept secret. If male partners find out, they may leave seropositive women, abuse them emotionally or physically, or even murder them. At least two women have been shot for their seropositivity and "many others" have been injured (*Baltimore Sun* 10/14/93).

PREVENTION IMPLICATIONS

Risk reduction among HIV-positive people is called **secondary prevention**. Secondary prevention helps protect already ill individuals from further health insults by keeping germs that could otherwise be transmitted during sexual interaction (or injectable drug use) from entering their bodies. It also helps contain HIV. Risk reduction undertaken by uninfected people is called **primary prevention**.

Research has shown that building cultural awareness and gender sensitivity into AIDS education and intervention programs can make them more effective. As Bolton and Singer point out:

Prevention works best when it promotes change through individual and community empowerment strategies informed by holistic understandings of the local context, when it acknowledges the positive contributions of local cultural values to the process of change, and when it incorporates an array of options that permit individuals to transform their lives in ways that enhance their physical, emotional, and material well-being. Prevention efforts fail when they revictimize and stigmatize those who do not accept messages incompatible with their basic values and needs, when they blame those whose behavior suggests recalcitrance or relapse from risk standards established by health "experts," when they are based on top-down rather than community designed and implemented approaches, and when they are shaped by the moralistic and authoritarian models. (Bolton and Singer 1992: 4; italics in original)

The more kinds of interventions offered in a given community (e.g., street outreach, clinic counseling, community-center meetings, etc.)—and the more involved community members are in shaping these interventions—the more chance of success educators will have. The importance of maintaining a sensitivity to local cultural values is paramount. Approaches to AIDS education that both glorify monogamy and offer condom advice for the nonmonogamous ("bad" people) undermine themselves. In cultures that promote monogamy, as mainstream American culture does, optimistic bias leads people to cast themselves as monogamous ("good" people), therefore having no need for protection.

In order to encourage, rather than discourage, the practice of safer sex, educators need to recognize the particular aspects of a group's feelings and ideas about condoms and sexual relationships that can be productively appealed to. For example, in cultures that hold relationship ideals recommending faithful monogamy, educators might cast condom use as an act of altruistic love and commitment rather than an identity-threatening admission of current sexual unfaithfulness.

The link between altruism and risk-reduction could be advantageously used. Research has shown that educational promotions directed to men will be more successful if they "portray clearly the health risks that unprotected intercourse creates for women and children" (457). For example, as anthropologist Keith Bletzer explains, "The AIDS educator can incorporate a discussion of male responsibility to women as another aspect of 'being a man'" (1993: 16); that is, the cultural definition of manhood can be exploited. If a spouse's or child's health already has been affected, grief may provide motivation to reduce risk-taking behavior among men if sensitive intervention is provided (Nyamathi, Shuler, and Porche 1990).

It is not enough to sell condoms as symbols of love and care when the loving, caring act of condom use is still presented or perceived as a bother and a chore. AIDS educators inadvertently encourage clients to hold onto (or, in some cases, to develop) anticondom sentiments by portraying condoms as disruptive and bothersome. Condom use can be portrayed as an integral part of sexual interaction. It is a skill that is learned; without good skills, it can be problematic (Thompson, Yager, and Martin 1993). Further, without lubricant—and many of the condoms that clinics provide for free are dry—sex with condoms can be quite painful for the partner receiving penetration.

Sex-positive information on how condoms can enhance sex (e.g., by making erections last longer) and instruction on how to incorporate condoms into the sex act pleasurably should be a regular part of AIDS interventions. Tanner and Pollack (1988) found that couples who received eroticized and sex-positive instructions on condom use had significantly enhanced attitudes toward condoms. Bletzer (1993) found that Latino migrant workers consider the act of penetrative sexual intercourse to be natural and cleansing; sex-positive cultural ideas such as this can be built upon in education programs.

In addition to condoms, the promotion of which suggests that penetrative-receptive intercourse involving the penis is the only legitimate form of sex, alternative safer-sex strategies should be promoted. As Taylor and

Lourea contend, "It is much easier for people to increase sexual options than to extinguish established patterns" (1992: 107).

While improved interventions will help increase condom-use rates, they are not the only answer. Impoverished people and members of disenfranchised minority groups also need better access to health care services, which will lead to better overall health. Better health will make it harder for HIV to gain a foothold in the body, and improved health care delivery will lead individuals to become more trusting of the system's AIDS prevention recommendations. Those most vulnerable to AIDS also are those who need improved educational and employment opportunities. As Anitra Pivnick suggests, employment can "generate feelings of accomplishment, independence, and personal worth" (1993: 449). Such feelings can enhance a person's interest in, and ability to insist on, safer sex.

Safer-sex promotions often take place one-on-one in the clinic setting. But health care providers and educators can apply numerous effective techniques, including group sessions and using more comfortable and familiar settings such as churches, homes, and even bars. The participation of community members can also be encouraged to increase credibility and to reach people who would otherwise fall through the cracks, such as homeless people and drug addicts.

Using mixed gender groups could lead to better intergender understanding, thereby helping to clear up misconceptions that the genders have about each other. For example, men might not actually have such negative views about condoms as women think they do (Kegeles, Adler, and Irwin 1988; Schoenborn, Marsh, and Hardy 1994). Knowledge of this might make women less hesitant to suggest condom use.

Community and group outreach is also conducive to combating AIDS-related myths, such as that AIDS was invented by the army as part of a germ-warfare scheme, or clear up misconceptions that mosquitoes can spread HIV. To dismiss such notions out of hand could validate clients' beliefs that the health care system does not care about them and cannot be trusted (DeParle 1990; Herek and Capitanio 1994). Common-sense beliefs must therefore be fought with respectful, common-sense logic.

Another thought problem that educators might address concerns condoms' contraceptive function; using condoms when one or both sex partners has undergone sterilization or when another family planning method is used can seem redundant. Clients need to be reminded that condoms serve as barriers for HIV and other STDs in addition to being useful for family planning, and they therefore lower the chances that a later planned-for baby will contract AIDS.

As the example of AIDS shows us, in order to promote education, positive attitudes, healthy behaviors, and effective care, it is essential to consider, understand, and utilize the connections between social and cultural factors in illness and care. This requires an integrated approach to the human experience of health and illness, as well as an expansion of the biomedical model.

INTEGRATION OF HEALTH CARE MODALITIES

Many factors block such expansion and integration. Probably one of the strongest barriers to integration is the primacy of the scientific model, which, even with its limitations, is necessary and vital. Without it, we would have no progress or advance through technology and no real understanding of biological and physical processes.

The scientific method's record is extremely impressive with discoveries in genetics, advances in diagnostic and surgical technology, improvements in acute care, and better quality and extension of life. Due to the strong focus on the scientific aspect of biomedicine, however, there has been, until recently, very little research demonstrating the efficacy or benefits of non-biomedical therapeutic interventions, either alone or in combination with biomedical treatments, and only limited attempts at incorporation of alternative values or care into care regimens.

Prejudice, distrust, and competition between both biomedical and alternative practitioners are certainly additional factors. Some biomedical practitioners may only be interested in a one-way process of cooptation. Sometimes, plans to bring competing systems under control may be initiated only in order to bring more people into the biomedical system proper with no real understanding of what other systems may offer in terms of care and treatment.

Despite the many problems, possibilities of integration cannot be dismissed, nor can we assume the outcome will be negative. Integration of modalities can yield some very positive results.

SUCCESSFUL INTEGRATION

Joint Collaboration

While most success stories have not yet happened, one is by now an anthropological classic. That is the story of the Navajo-Cornell Medical School joint project (Adair, Deuschle, and Barnett 1988). In this project, anthropologists John Adair and Clifford Barnett joined physician Kurt Deuschle to design and administer an experimental health program on the Navajo reservation in Arizona. The project, initiated in the early 1950s, was carried out in partnership with the Navajo Tribal Council and the Tribal Health Committee, chaired by Annie Wauneka. From the beginning, contact between all parties was respectful and honest. The project was jointly funded (the Tribal Council had contributed $10,000 1953 dollars);

ownership and all that it entails—including responsibility, accountability, and pride in a job well done—was jointly distributed.

Cultural sensitivity infused the project and fueled its appeal. Initial discussions concerned tuberculosis, which had been a major problem on the reservation, affecting one in ten Navajo after World War II (Adair, Deuschle, and Barnett 1988: 19). The area to be served was selected by the Tribal Health Committee, and the citizens of the area, called the Many Farms-Rough Rock district, were asked by the health committee to support the project. The clinic was blessed by a medicine man on its opening day. So, from its inception, the clinic enjoyed local support and promised to address pressing local needs rather than what insiders defined as nonproblems.

One of the keys to the success of the Many Farms project was the fact that project workers were committed to spending time "ascertaining which of the native institutions are still vital and highly valued in their present form" (Adair, Deuschle, and Barnett 1988: 109). Clinicians built local forms of social organization into medical record keeping practices, for example, by recording clanship (119). In addition, native practitioners were consulted for ideas and opinions from the initial days of the project's inception. Of course, from the Navajo point of view, the clinic was incorporated by native medical practitioners such that traditional and biomedical systems became integrated.

To diagnose illness, Navajo shamans go into trance and practice hand trembling, in which hand movements produce various designs in the sand that are then interpreted or read. After the clinic's establishment, native diagnosticians could, on the basis of the signs, refer patients to the clinic just as they could, on the basis of the signs, recommend particular traditional healing strategies or even recommend that the patient combine both types of response. Of the forty-nine native practitioners in the area, only three had not visited the clinic themselves (Adair, Deuschle, and Barnett 1988: 167). Many clinic patients utilized both medical systems, and the project clinicians never discouraged this; some Navajo clinic workers had themselves been trained in traditional healing ways (e.g., 91).

The integration of the two systems was facilitated by native notions about ill health. The Navajo feel that there are some diseases (e.g., tuberculosis) that biomedicine is simply better suited to cure. Likewise, others are best diagnosed and treated with native techniques (e.g., sickness caused by getting too close to a spot in which lightening has struck). And some, such as snake bites, are treated equally well by either system (Adair, Deuschle, and Barnett 1988: 163). Because Navajo do not feel that their medicine is all-powerful, room can easily be made for biomedicine, respectfully practiced.

Clinic clients interviewed said that when symptom onset was sudden and pain acute, they would first seek clinic assistance. But when onset was slow or pain lingered, or when the problem entailed general malaise, help was first sought from a native practitioner (Adair, Deuschle, and Barnett 1988: 169). Of 100 Many Farms clinic patients interviewed between 1961 and 1962, eighty-two had seen a native healer before visiting the clinic; three-fourths of the fifty-eight patients in the sample with acute conditions saw a native healer after their clinic visits (Adair, Deuschle, and Barnett 1988: 168). The integration of treatment modalities by clients reflected their view that each system performed a different function and that these functions had to be performed at different times (first or second) for different conditions.

In the words of Adair and his colleagues, this integration reflects "a recognition that illness in the individual involves many components needing treatment and both systems are necessary for complete treatment" (1988: 170). So, for example, a medicine man with appendicitis had a healing ceremony performed after his appendectomy. He explained that the ceremony would help the incision to heal. Further, it provided a ritualized means of reentering his community after the hospital stay; his relatives, neighbors, and friends attended the ceremony, wished him well, and expressed pleasure at his presence back home.

As the Many Farms project was an experiment related initially to tuberculosis abatement, it eventually was terminated. However, as the project leaders wrote in 1988, "In the years since the closing of the Many Farms Clinic the Navajo people have made considerable progress in taking over the administration of their own public health programming, especially in the areas of health education and prevention" (241). In addition to simple sensitivity to cultural differences and respect for native ways, the emphasis of the project on direct Navajo participation accounts to a large degree for the project's success.

Integration of Biomedicine with Community

As the collaborative Navajo example shows, the need to expand the role of biomedical practitioners, especially those in primary care, does not actually entail an impossible work load or extended study and responsibility. Practitioners are already politically oriented through professional interests. As they interact with families and communities, the workload entailed by cultural sensitivity may be shared, and such sharing may improve relationships and mutual understanding among clients and practitioners. The term "patient advocate" thereby becomes more meaningful and patients may also become "practitioner advocates."

The concept of health and illness, in addition, must be expanded to include culturally relevant definitions that are demonstrably related to treatment outcomes. As demonstrated in chapter 2, many health problems are linked to poverty and social and environmental conditions such that curative medical treatment provides only a momentary palliative. For example, a child's rash might clear up with ointment. But if the rash is caused by exposure to some kind of toxin in the child's play environment, and the toxin is not removed from that environment, the rash will keep reappearing. The old saying that "An ounce of prevention is worth a pound of cure" speaks to this problem. In many cases, the ounce of prevention needed has to do with improving life environments through the development of community resources, including education, provision of services, and community empowerment.

This point is clearly seen in a brief review of some of the work of Caroll Behrhorst, a Kansas physician who worked for nearly thirty years in Guatemala; his work there relates to problems of health care delivery in parts of the United States. Behrhorst (now deceased) founded a small clinic and teaching center in Chimaltenango. In addition to on-site and outreach health work, carried out by local people trained by Behrhorst, the center also instituted agricultural development programs with the aim of increasing people's living standards and self-sufficiency.

As Behrhorst tells it, his emphasis on **community development** grew from a realization that "I was trying to empty an ocean of disease and malfunction with a medical teaspoon" (1993: 58). After treating children suffering from malaise, puffy eyes, swollen feet, discolorations of the skin, diarrhea, and coughing, Behrhorst "realized that, no matter how many times we treated [the youngsters], they would never be healthy until basic changes were made in the village" (58).

The changes "began in a simple, tentative way" (Behrhorst 1993: 60), when a Peace Corps volunteer working in the clinic who had gained the trust of people living in Chimaltenango and the surrounding villages began to introduce new farming methods. Later, some money was lent from the clinic's operating funds to allow a group of twenty-five village families to invest in laying chickens. Soon, people had more protein in their diets. Moreover, they had more faith in their own abilities. Another group borrowed money to buy some land, and another formed a weaving and marketing cooperative. As cash began to flow, the loans were repaid. The health of the villagers improved dramatically once they had a firm economic base to sustain them. As Behrhorst wrote, "What started as curing the sick broadened into a general community program geared to activities that the residents want and need and that result in self-empowerment" (60–61).

All along, Behrhorst and the local people worked to make the clinic independent both in terms of staffing and finances, rather than allowing the Chimaltenango project to remain dependent on outside aid. Nurses, doctors, and other staff who are outsiders may stay for only a few years or months before leaving a clinic. Further, financial aid is not always reliable and may have strings attached. Behrhorst said, "If we outsiders do not plan ways of doing ourselves out of a job we are probably not doing the job at all" (1993: 61). In 1975, the Chimaltenango project was identified by the World Health Organization (WHO) as one of ten worldwide models for effective health promotion, and later WHO declarations and agendas were built to a large degree on the model Behrhorst and his Guatemalan colleagues had developed (Luecke 1993: xviii).

Similar programs have since been put into place in the United States. For example, people living in a predominantly poor black community on the west side of Chicago formed a voluntary community organization in the mid–1970s to address health problems. Their struggles and triumphs are described by John McKnight (1993).

The first problem confronted was that of a lack of access to local hospitals. After this hurdle was surmounted and both employment in and access to the services of the two local hospitals increased, the health status of community members still did not improve. Hospital medical records revealed that the main health problems of the community were not, in fact, the kinds that are best solved through curative medicine.

The most common reasons for the hospitalization of community members were, in order of frequency, automobile accidents, interpersonal attacks, accidents (other than those involving autos), bronchial ailments, alcoholism, drug-related problems, and dog bites. McKnight writes,

The people of the organization were startled by these findings. . . . The medicalization of health had led them to believe that the hospitals were appropriately addressing their health problems, but they discovered instead that the hospitals were dealing with many problems for which hospitals are always too late and which required treatment of another sort. It was an important step in the health consciousness of this community to recognize that modern medical systems are frequently dealing with maladies that are social problems rather than diseases. (1993: 221)

After considering their options, the people in the organization decided to start at the bottom of the list. Dog bites accounted for about 4 percent of all emergency room visits. Dogs were indeed a neighborhood nuisance; packs of wild dogs had recently taken up residence in the area. The organization let it be known through neighborhood block associations that they would pay a bounty or reward for each captured dog. The neighborhood youth thought this a great game, and in one month's time 160 dogs were captured. Emergency room admissions for dog bites went down accordingly. Not only had the group learned that their own actions could improve health, but they also were involving community youth in positive, community-building activities.

After their initial success, the group targeted automobile accidents for reduction. They first sought to find out where most accidents occurred. The group turned to city planners. They plotted three months' worth of figures on a map of the neighborhood to locate the most dangerous areas. In one 60-foot-wide area, six people had been injured and one killed. This area was the entrance to a department store. The organization contacted the owner of the department store and successfully negotiated for a change in the way that the entrance was laid out.

Bronchial problems were the third issue addressed by the community health organization. The group learned that such problems were linked to nutrition and concluded that people in the neighborhood did not eat enough fresh fruit and vegetables. They could not afford to. Several members of the group noted that greenhouses might be built on top of the flat roofs of neighborhood dwellings. And, as McKnight recalls, "a number of fascinating things began to happen" (1993: 224).

The greenhouses worked: they provided inexpensive fruit and vegetables. People saw that in addition to simply providing them with good things to eat, the greenhouses also could provide commodities that they could sell to generate income. Further, the greenhouses, sitting atop people's dwellings, served as insulation and absorbed heat that might otherwise have leaked out of the rooftops.

The community organization owned a retirement home for the elderly. One day, one of the residents wandered into the greenhouse. She started to work there on a regular basis. Other residents joined her there. According to the home's administrator, the attitude of these residents changed. McKnight recalls that "They were excited. They had found a function and a purpose. The greenhouse had become a tool to empower the elderly—it enabled discarded people to become productive" (1993: 225).

Overall, the group's mission involved removing the underlying causes of disease or injury when they could, and adding health-promoting options into the community when possible. McKnight explains, "Converting medical problems into community issues proved central to health improvement [and] increased the organization's vitality and power" (1993: 226). The health actions instigated led away from overdependence on the local hospital and toward self-sufficient or low-consumption health strategies. In light of the ever-increasing costs of providing clinical care, and the increasing fragmentation of communities throughout the United States, the promotion of similar groups' health and community building activities seems a sound investment.

Sociocultural Medicine?

Anthropologist Robert Hahn recently offered the following proposition:

If the healing process invariably requires an understanding of different perceptions of the world; if understandings of sickness are culturally given and organized; if sickness is caused in part by social organization and social relations; if healing depends on effective relationships across cultural boundaries; if, in other words, social and cultural conditions and events underlie the healing process, then healers—biomedical and other—unwittingly make anthropological assumptions about themselves, their patients, and their interactions in the course of medical practice. (Hahn 1995: 268–69)

As Hahn humbly states in his review of the literature on biomedical practice, he is not the first to observe that this is so. However, he is among the first to make a powerful argument for the institutionalization of what he terms "anthropological medicine." Anthropological medicine, Hahn explains,

is a theory and practice that gives primacy to sickness—conditions of patients as conceived as unwanted by themselves—that accepts the social and cultural roots of both professional and lay ideas and attitudes of sickness; that fully recognizes the etiology of sickness in social and cultural as well as physiological and environmental conditions, that also acknowledges sociocultural effects in therapy and healing processes and respects the social context of healing. . . . It integrates a sociocultural perspective with a biological one at the core of medical education, medical practice, research, and institutional arrangements. (Hahn 1995: 265–66)

In effect, Hahn argues that because medicine is at heart cross-cultural—because patients and healers always bring (at least slightly and sometimes wildly) different ideas with them to their clinical encounters—"an anthropological perspective is a basic and essential component of good medical theory and practice rather than a peripheral, optional one" (1995: 266). Listening, understanding sociocultural context, and recognizing intraethnic variability are key principles of medicine in Hahn's view. Good practice also depends on explaining, translating, and brokering between cultural worlds and respecting, responding to, and accommodating others' needs and desires.

Hahn's point about intraethnic variability merits additional comment here. Throughout this book, we have included examples from across many cultural and social contexts. We have sometimes drawn attention to syndromes that occur most commonly in specific cultural contexts or that people from given cultures attend to, such as *susto, empacho, high blood,* and *high-pertension.* We have done so in an effort to bring some life and immediacy to the theoretical concepts we are attempting to teach. However, we have made a complementary effort not to suggest that particular formulas for ethnic or cultural sensitivity be followed in constructing clinical care regimens, but rather to argue that flexibility be maintained and skills developed in cultural assessment by the care giver, which takes into account the individual client's expressed or perceived needs (Hahn 1995; Majumdar 1995).

THE CALL FOR NEW PARADIGMS

There has been much recognition of the need for new or expanded paradigms for the delivery of health and medical care. We argue that any new paradigm must consider and include cultural diversity and its additional dimensions and therapies in prevention, diagnosis, and treatment. Science is vital, but its interpretations and applications have become inadequate to meet the challenges faced by the health care system. Ultimate solutions must be located within the human condition, with additional focus on cultural aspects and diversity, and on individual *and* social responsibility.

In 1991, only 23 percent of medical schools included family issues in the curriculum, only 24 percent taught about the biopsychosocial model, only 17 percent had instruction on cultural differences, and only 17 percent taught interpersonal skills (Novack 1993: 291). The full institutionalization and utilization of anthropological and sociological theory and practice by the dominant medical system will "demand a reorientation of current practice" and will require "substantial revisions" in the ways in which health professionals are trained (Novack 1993).

MULTICULTURALISM REVISITED

As the United States moves in a direction of even greater diversity, with 47 percent of the population estimated to be black, Hispanic, or Asian by the year 2050 (U.S. Bureau of the Census 1993b), the debate over multiculturalism will undoubtedly intensify. The attacks on multiculturalism (Schlesinger 1992; Bennett 1992; Bloom 1987) stem from a concern over power and privilege, and the same might be said of attacks on the diversity of health-related cultural systems and perceptions (an alternative response is found in Levine 1996).

The biomedical model, long associated with core American values and superiority, is not designed to meet the human challenges of social and technological change. New strategies and philosophies must be incorporated within the health delivery system to meet the challenges, focused on links and interrelationships, rather than supremacy of one sector over others.

Health care is becoming more multicultural and pluralistic. Providers, as well as patients, now come from increasingly diverse backgrounds. Women and minorities are moving steadily into the field of medicine. Because of demographic trends, "older adults, including the 'baby boomers,' will be cared for by large numbers of health care professionals who are people of color, and will be financially supported by the taxes of large numbers of younger people of color" (Feagin, Vera, and Zsembik 1996: 17).

The application of multiculturalism in health care is neither "un-American" nor unreasonable. The orientation of biomedicine's service to suffering humanity should not distinguish or select to whom that service will be given. The art of medicine is the art of human relationships and communication and, most of all, caring. There is a growing recognition, even among biomedical providers, that complementary medicine may expand the resources for both caring and curing.

Biomedicine is not acultural. It must respond to changing needs and expectations as part of an expanding multicultural world. Feagin, Vera, and Zsembik point out that many of the ethnic and other conflicts in the world are generated by the demand for economic, political, and social recognition and power: "The unique identities of individuals can be respected only when each group and culture is fully respected and equally influential. Diversity is thus coterminous with real democracy" (1996: 19). The challenge is there for all of us.

FOR DISCUSSION

1. What are the barriers to health care encountered by impoverished minority women? How do these compare to the barriers encountered by impoverished minority men, by recent immigrants, and by gays?

2. How did modernization contribute to the spread of AIDS? How does sexism contribute to the spread of AIDS? How does racism contribute?

3. What impact can AIDS have on families? How will this vary cross-culturally?

4. Discuss the impact that the association between AIDS and homosexuality and drug use has had on the public's response to the disease.

5. Try to identify some of the means and methods of integration that already exist in health care delivery in the United States. Can you find examples of resistance and separation? To what extent can integration take place, and how can we bridge the gaps?

6. How can we promote cultural diversity in health care, and what are some common human strengths we can also promote?

Appendix: Resources for Cultural Assessment and Achieving Cultural Sensitivity

I. USEFUL REFERENCES FOR MULTICULTURAL CARE

Adair, J., K. Deuschle, and C. Barnett. 1988. *The People's Health: Anthropology and Medicine in a Navajo Community*. Revised and Expanded. Albuquerque: University of New Mexico Press.

Cormier, L., W. Cormier, and R. Weisser. 1984. *Interviewing and Helping Skills for Health Professionals*. Monterey, CA: Wadsworth Health Sciences.

Fuller, J., and P. Toon. 1988. *Medical Practice in a Multicultural Society*. London: Heinemann.

Galanti, G. 1991. *Caring for Patients from Different Cultures: Case Studies from American Hospitals*. Philadelphia: University of Pennsylvania Press.

Helman, C. 1995. *Culture, Health and Illness*. 3rd ed. London: Butterworth-Heinemann.

Julia, M. 1996. *Multicultural Awareness in the Health Professions*. Needham Heights, MA: Allyn and Bacon.

Kavanagh, K., and P. Kennedy. 1992. *Promoting Cultural Diversity Strategies for Health Care Professionals*. Newbury Park, CA: Sage.

Kreps, G., and E. Kunimoto. 1994. *Effective Communication in Multicultural Health Settings*. Thousand Oaks, CA: Sage.

Locke, D. 1992. *Increasing Multicultural Understanding: A Comprehensive Model*. Newbury Park, CA: Sage.

Luecke, R., ed. 1993. *A New Dawn in Guatemala: Toward a Worldwide Health Vision*. Prospect Heights, IL: Waveland Press.

Majumdar, B. 1995. *Culture and Health: Culture-Sensitive Training Manual for the Health Care Provider*, 4th ed. Hamilton, Ontario: McMaster University.

Pedersen, P., and D. Hernandez. 1996. *Decisional Interviewing in a Cultural Context.* Thousand Oaks, CA: Sage.

Seelye, H., ed. 1996. *Experiential Activities for Intercultural Learning.* Vol. 1. Yarmouth, ME: Intercultural Press.

Shepherd, J., ed. 1994. *Violence in Health Care: A Practical Guide to Coping with Violence and Caring for Victims.* New York: Oxford University Press.

Straus, M., ed. 1988. *Abuse and Victimization Across the Life Span.* Baltimore: Johns Hopkins University Press.

2. SOME PROJECT SUGGESTIONS RELATED TO AIDS EDUCATION

These exercises have been built around HIV/AIDS. However, other health problems, such as tobacco use, hypertension, or breast or prostate cancer, could easily be substituted. These questions and issues can also be used to develop problems for problem-based learning exercises as discussed below in section 5.

1. Design a condom promotion program for a minority group living in your town. What cultural factors would have to be kept in mind? What socioeconomic factors and what gender factors would need to be considered?

2. Test the strength of the optimistic bias in your class. With the help of your instructor, design a survey to measure how "at risk" people feel. Do they feel that their chances of HIV infection are high or low? Why? How do they compare their own risks with those of most of their peers? (You might include a number of groups here: best friends, classmates, neighbors, people your age nationally, etc.) On what basis is that comparison made? Ask a class that has not studied AIDS in depth, as you have, to complete the survey, too. How do the classes' answers compare? What might explain any differences?

3. Survey two weeks' worth of newspapers for AIDS-related stories. Examine these stories for bias. What patterns emerge? How do they relate to cultural understandings or social processes? (Different groups of students in your class might be assigned to monitor different kinds of media: music magazines, science magazines, beauty and body magazines, national newspapers, local newspapers, tabloids, etc.)

4. Observe behavior in the condom section of a supermarket or drugstore for two hours. (It might be a good idea to let the manager know that you are doing a class project.) What walks of life did customers come from (and who seemed to be missing)? How did these people seem to handle their selections? What barriers or facilitators did they seem to encounter? How might price or selling practices have come into play?

3. MAJOR WEB SITES FOR RELATED TOPICS

American Holistic Medicine Association
http://www.doubleclickd.com

Centers for Disease Control and Prevention
http://www.cdc.gov

Health Professionals for Diversity
http://www.aamc.org

Health World
http://www.healthy.net/

Martindales' Health Science Guide
http://www-sci.lib.uci.edu/HSG/HSGuide.html

Medical Education Online (journal)
http://www.utmb.edu/meo/

National Institutes of Health (NIH)
http://www.nih.gov

National Institute of Mental Health
http://www.nimh.nih.gov

Society for Medical Anthropology
http://www.people.memphis.edu/~sma

Williams & Wilkins webROUNDS (on-line medical student journal)
http://www.wwilkins.com/rounds

The World Health Organization
http://www.who.Ch/Welcome.html

4. ADDITIONAL SOURCES FOR MULTICULTURAL TRAINING

Videos

May be purchased from Insight Media, 2162 Broadway, New York, NY 10024:

"Communication Skills in a Multicultural World"
(1994/ 20 min./#EP213)

"Cross-Cultural Communication in Diverse Settings"
(1992/ 60 min./#EP53)

"Valuing Diversity: Multicultural Communication"
(1994/ 49 min./#EP246)

From the Center for Health Care Ethics, 440 S. Batavia, Orange, CA 92668:

"Ethical Perceptions of Men and Women: Are They Different?"
(11 min.)

Journals or Newsletters

Alternative Therapies in Health and Medicine

Anthropology and Medicine

Complementary Medicine for the Physician (newsletter), from Churchill Livingstone, Inc.

Health: An Interdisciplinary Journal for the Social Study of Health, Illness and Medicine

The Journal of Alternative and Complementary Medicine

The Journal of Health and Social Behavior

Medical Anthropology

Medical Anthropology Quarterly

Social Science and Medicine

5. PROBLEM-BASED LEARNING: A STUDENT-CENTERED TECHNIQUE

An excellent technique for learning about cultural issues in health care is problem-based learning, a technique being adopted by a number of medical schools and other teaching institutions. The technique is different from conventional teaching, in that the role of teacher becomes one of facilitator, while learning is centered on the students. Learning results from the group process when students work together to understand or resolve a given problem scenario, using joint collaboration in brain-storming, identifying related issues, and doing research and evaluation of various facets of the problem, including possible resolutions. Students thus become responsible for their own learning, guided by the teacher. Information about and instructions for use of the technique can be found in:

Barrows, H., and R. Tamblyn, 1980. *Problem-based Learning: An Approach to Medical Education.* New York: Springer.
Schmidt, H., W. Dauphinee, and V. Patel. 1987. "Comparing the Effects of Problem-based Learning and Conventional Curricula in an International Sample." *Journal of Medical Education* 62:305–15.
Wilkerson, L., and G. Feletti. 1989. "Problem-based Learning: One Approach to Increasing Student Participation." In *The Department Chairperson's Role in Enhancing College Teaching, New Directions for Teaching and Learning,* edited by A. Lucas, 51–60. San Francisco: Jossey-Bass.

Bibliography

Abelove, H. 1994. "The Politics of the 'Gay Plague': AIDS as a U.S. Ideology." In *Body Politics: Disease, Desire, and the Family*, edited by M. Ryan and A. Gordon, 3–17. San Francisco: Westview Press.

Abraham, L. 1997. "The Myth of the Sexist Doc." *Health* 11(6):72–80.

Adair, J., K. Deuschle, and C. Barnett. 1988. *The People's Health: Anthropology and Medicine in a Navajo Community*, rev. and expanded. Albuquerque: University of New Mexico Press.

Adams, P., and V. Benson. 1991. *Current Estimates from the National Health Interview Survey*. Hyattsville, MD: National Center for Health Statistics, Vital and Health Statistics. 10:181.

AIDS Alert. 1993. "Research Gaining Support for Vaginal Microbicide." *AIDS Alert* 8(9):134.

American Medical Association. 1993 edition and previous editions. *Physician Characteristics and Distribution in the U.S.* Chicago: Survey and Data Resources, American Medical Association.

Anderson, E. 1990. *Streetwise: Race, Class, and Change in an Urban Neighborhood*. Chicago: University of Chicago Press.

Annas, G. 1994. "Women, Health Care, and the Law: Birth, Death, and In Between." In *An Unfinished Revolution: Women and Health Care in America*, edited by E. Friedman, 29–45. New York: United Hospital Fund of New York.

Arellano, R., and S. Kearny. 1992. *Cultural Considerations (A Supplement to Teaching Hospital: Cultural Determinants of Health and Illness and Their Importance in Effective Health-Care Delivery at University Hospital)*. Albuquerque: Creative Services/Dissemination Unit of the Health of the Public Program, University of New Mexico School of Medicine.

Aries, P. 1974. *Western Attitudes Toward Death: From the Middle Ages to the Present*. Baltimore: Johns Hopkins University Press.

Armstrong, D. 1987. "Theoretical Tensions in Biopsychosocial Medicine." *Social Science and Medicine* 25(11):1213–18.

———. 1989. *An Outline of Sociology as Applied to Medicine*. 3rd ed. London: Wright.

Atchley, R. 1994. *Social Forces and Aging: An Introduction to Gerontology*, 7th ed. Belmont, CA: Wadsworth.

Atkinson, P. 1978. "From Honey to Vinegar: Levi-Strauss in Vermont." In *Culture and Curing: Anthropological Perspectives*, edited by P. Morley and R. Wallis. Pittsburgh: University of Pittsburgh Press.

Augé, M., and C. Herzlich, eds. 1995 [1983]. *The Meaning of Illness: Anthropology, History and Sociology*, translated from the French by K. Durnin, C. Lambein, K. Leclercq-Jones, B. Garnier, and R. Williams. London: Harwood Academic Publishers.

Baer, H. 1989. "The American Dominative Medical System as a Reflection of Social Relations in the Larger Society." *Social Science and Medicine* 28(11):1103–12.

Baer, R. 1996. "Mental Health Among Mexican-Americans: Implications for Survey Research." *Human Organization* 55(1):58–66.

Baltimore Sun. 1993, (10/14). "Women with AIDS Risk Assault by Partners," p. 16A.

Barnes, B. 1985. *About Science*. New York: Basil Blackwell.

Bart, P. 1969. "Why Women's Status Changes with Middle Age." *Sociological Symposium*, No. 3. Blacksburg, VA: VPI and State University, Department of Sociology.

Becker, A. 1994. "Nurturing and Negligence: Working on Others' Bodies in Fiji." In *Embodiment and Experience: The Existential Ground of Culture and Self*, edited by T. Csordas, 100–115. Cambridge: Cambridge University Press.

Becker, M., ed. 1974. *The Health Belief Model and Personal Health Behavior*. San Francisco: Society for Public Health Education.

Becker, M., and L. Maiman. 1975. *The Health Belief Model and Personal Health Behavior*. San Francisco: Society for Public Health Education.

Beckford, J. 1984. "Holistic Imagery and Ethics in New Religious and Healing Movements." *Social Compass* 21(2–3):259–72.

Beckman, H., K. Markakis, A. Suchman, and R. Frankel. 1994. "The Doctor-Patient Relationship and Malpractice: Lessons from Plaintiff Depositions." *Archives of Internal Medicine* 154:1365–70.

Behrhorst, C. 1993. "The Chimaltenango Development Program." In *A New Dawn in Guatemala: Toward a Worldwide Health Vision*, edited by R. Luecke, 55–76. Prospect Heights, IL: Waveland Press.

Bennett, W. 1992. *The De-Valuing of America: The Fight for Our Culture and Our Children*. New York: Summit Books.

Berliner, H. 1975. "A Larger Perspective on the Flexner Report." *International Journal of Health Services* 5(4):573–92.

Berliner, H., and J. Salmon. 1980. "The Holistic Alternative to Scientific Medicine:

History and Analysis." *International Journal of Health Services* 10(1):133–47.

Bernard, H. R. 1994. *Research Methods in Anthropology: Qualitative and Quantitative Approaches*, 2nd ed. Walnut Creek, CA: AltaMira Press.

Bettelheim, B. 1962 [1954]. *Symbolic Wounds: Puberty Rites and the Envious Male*. New York: Collier Books.

Bezemer, W. 1992. "Women and HIV." *Journal of Psychology and Human Sexuality* 5(1, 2):31–36.

Bhatia, J., D. Vir, A. Timmappaya, and C. Chuttani. 1975. "Traditional Healers and Modern Medicine." *Social Science and Medicine* 9(1):15–21.

Bletzer, K. 1993. "Migrant HIV Education in the Wake of the AIDS Crisis." *Practicing Anthropology* 15(4):13–16.

Bloom, A. 1987. *The Closing of the American Mind*. New York: Simon and Schuster.

Bodeker, G. 1996. "Global Health Traditions." In *Fundamentals of Complementary and Alternative Medicine*, edited by M. Micozzi, 279–90. New York: Churchill Livingstone.

Bollini, P. 1995. "Health and Mental Health Among Mexican-American Migrants: Implications for Survey Research." *World Health* 48(6):20–21.

Bolton, R. 1992. "AIDS and Promiscuity: Muddles in the Models." In *Rethinking AIDS Prevention*, edited by R. Bolton and M. Singer, 7–85. New York: Gordon and Breach Science Publishers.

Bolton, R., and M. Singer. 1992. "Introduction. Rethinking HIV Prevention: Critical Assessments of the Content and Delivery of AIDS Risk-Reduction Messages." In *Rethinking AIDS Prevention*, edited by R. Bolton and M. Singer, 1–5. New York: Gordon and Breach Science Publishers.

Borden, W. 1991. "Beneficial Outcomes in Adjustment to HIV Seropositivity." *Social Service Review* 65(3):434–49.

Bordo, S. 1993. *Unbearable Weight: Feminism, Western Culture, and the Body*. Los Angeles: University of California Press.

Brandt, A. 1991. "Emerging Themes in the History of Medicine." *The Milbank Quarterly* 69(2):199–214.

Brink, P. J. 1989. "The Fattening Room Among the Annang of Nigeria." *Medical Anthropology* 12:131–43.

Broverman, J., D. Broverman, F. Clarkson, P. Rosenkrantz, and S. Vogel. 1970. "Sex-Role Stereotypes and Clinical Judgments of Mental Health." *Journal of Consulting and Clinical Psychiatry* 34(1):1–7.

Brown, E. 1979. *Rockefeller Medicine Men*. Berkeley: University of California Press.

Brown, P. 1995. "Naming and Framing: The Social Construction of Diagnosis and Illness." *Journal of Health and Social Behavior* (Extra Issue):34–52.

Browner, C. 1983. "Male Pregnancy Symptoms in Urban Colombia." *American Ethnologist* 10(3):494–511.

Browner, C. 1985. "Traditional Techniques for Diagnosis, Treatment, and Control of Pregnancy in Cali, Colombia." In *Women's Medicine: A Cross-Cultural Study of Indigenous Fertility Regulation*, edited by L. Newman, 99–123. New Brunswick, NJ: Rutgers University Press.

Buckley, T., an A. Gottleib. 1988. *Blood Magic: The Anthropology of Menstruation*. Berkeley: University of California Press.

Campbell, C. 1990. "Women and AIDS." *Social Science and Medicine* 30(4):407–15.

Cassidy, C. 1991. "The Good Body: When Bigger is Better." *Medical Anthropology* 13:181–213.

Cassileth, B., E. Lusk, T. Strouse, and B. Bodenheimer. 1984. "Contemporary Unorthodox Treatments in Cancer Medicine: A Study of Patients, Treatments, and Practitioners." *Annals of Internal Medicine* 101:105–12.

CDC [Centers for Disease Control and Prevention]. 1993a. *HIV/AIDS Prevention* 4(2).

CDC [Centers for Disease Control and Prevention]. 1993b. *HIV/AIDS Surveillance Report* 5(2).

CDC [Centers for Disease Control and Prevention]. 1995. *HIV/AIDS Surveillance Report* 7(2).

Chadwick, B., and T. Heaton, eds. 1992. *Statistical Handbook on the American Family*. New York: Oryx Press.

Chase, A. 1973. *The Biological Imperatives*. Baltimore: Penguin Books.

Cheng, T., J. Savageua, A. Sattler, and T. DeWitt. 1993. "Confidentiality in Health Care: A Survey of Knowledge, Perceptions, and Attitudes Among High School Students." *Journal of the American Medical Association* 269(11): 1404–7.

Chrisman, N. 1977. "The Health Seeking Process: An Approach to the Natural History of Illness." *Culture, Medicine and Psychiatry* 1:351–77.

Clark, J., D. Potter, and J. McKinlay. 1991. "Bringing Social Structure Back into Clinical Decision Making." *Social Science and Medicine* 8:853–66.

Clements, F. 1932. "Primitive Concepts of Disease." *University of California Publications in American Archaeology and Ethnology* 32:185–252.

Cochran, S. 1989. "Women and HIV Infection: Issues in Prevention and Behavioral Change." In *Primary Prevention of AIDS: Psychological Approaches*, edited by V. Mays, G. Albee, and S. Schneider, 309–27. Newbury Park, CA: Sage Publications.

Cockburn, A. 1963. *The Evolution and Eradication of Infectious Diseases*. Baltimore: Johns Hopkins University Press.

Cockerham, W. 1995. *Medical Sociology*, 6th ed. Englewood Cliffs, NJ: Prentice-Hall.

Coe, R. 1978. *Sociology of Medicine*. 2nd ed. New York: McGraw-Hill.

Coney, S. 1994. *The Menopause Industry: How the Medical Establishment Exploits Women*. U.S. ed., rev. Alameda, CA: Hunter House.

Conover, T. 1993. "Trucking Through the AIDS Belt: A Reporter at Large." *New Yorker* (August 16):56ff.

Conrad, P., and J. Schneider. 1992. *Deviance and Medicalization: From Badness to Sickness*, expanded ed. Philadelphia: Temple University Press.

Cook, R. 1972. *The Year of the Intern*. New York: The New American Library.

Corea, G. 1977. *The Hidden Malpractice: How American Medicine Mistreats Women*. New York: Jove/HBJ.

Corr, C., C. Nabe, and D. Corr. 1997. *Death and Dying, Life and Living*. 2nd ed. Pacific Grove, CA.: Brooks/Cole.

Cousins, N. 1979. *Anatomy of an Illness*. New York: W. W. Norton.

Cousins, N. 1981 [1979]. *Anatomy of an Illness as Perceived by the Patient: Reflections on Healing and Regeneration*. New York: Bantam Books.

Cowgill, D. 1972. *Aging and Modernization*. New York: Appleton-Century-Crofts.

Davis, D., and R. Whitten. 1987. "The Cross-Cultural Study of Human Sexuality." *Annual Reviews in Anthropology* 16:69–98.

Davis-Floyd, R. 1992. *Birth as an American Rite of Passage*. Los Angeles: University of California Press.

Demers, R., R. Altamore, H. Mustin, A. Kleinman, and D. Leonardi. 1980. "An Exploration of the Dimensions of Illness Behavior." *Journal of Family Practice* 11:1085–92.

DeParle, J. 1990. "Talk of Government Being Out to Get Blacks Falls on More Attentive Ears." *New York Times*, October 29, B-7.

Dietz, T. 1995. "Patterns of Intergenerational Assistance within the Mexican-American Family: Is the Family Taking Care of the Older Generations' Needs?" *Journal of Family Issues* 16(3):344–56.

DiMatteo, M., and D. DiNicola. 1982. *Achieving Patient Compliance: The Psychology of the Medical Practitioner's Role*. New York: Pergamon Press.

Dossey, L. 1982. *Space, Time and Medicine*. Boulder, CO: Shambhala Publications.

Dossey, L. 1991. *Meaning and Medicine*. New York: Bantam Books.

Dow, J. 1986. "Universal Aspects of Symbolic Meaning: A Theoretical Synthesis." *American Anthropologist* 88(1):56–69.

Dressler, W. 1990. "Culture, Stress and Disease." In *Medical Anthropology: Contemporary Theory and Method*, edited by T. Johnson and C. Sargent, 248–67. New York: Praeger.

Dutton, D. 1978. "Explaining the Low Use of Health Services by the Poor: Costs, Attitudes, or Delivery Systems?" *American Sociological Review* 43 (June): 348–68.

Eagan, A. 1994. "The Women's Health Movement and Its Lasting Impact." In *An Unfinished Revolution: Health Care in America*, edited by E. Friedman, 15–27. New York: United Hospital Fund of New York.

Eastman, K., and M. Loustaunau. 1987. "Reacting to the Medical Bureaucracy: Lay Midwifery as a Birthing Alternative." *Marriage and Family Review* 11(3–4):23–37.

Edgar, H. 1992. "Outside the Community." *Hastings Center Report* 22(6):32–35.

Eisenberg, D., R. Kessler, C. Foster, F. Norlock, D. Calkins, and T. Delbanco. 1993. "Unconventional Medicine in the United States: Prevalence, Costs, and Patterns of Use." *New England Journal of Medicine* 328(4):246–52.

Eisenberg, L., and A. Kleinman, eds. 1981. *The Relevance of Social Science for Medicine*. Dordrecht, Holland: D. Reidel Publishing Co.

Eisenbruch, M. 1984. "Cross-cultural Aspects of Bereavement. II: Ethnic and Cultural Variations in the Development of Bereavement Practices." *Culture, Medicine and Psychiatry* 8:315–47.

Emanuel, E., and L. Emanuel. 1992. "Four Models of the Physician-Patient Relationship." *Journal of the American Medical Association* 267(16):2221–6.

Engel G. 1977. "The Need for a New Medical Model: A Challenge for Biomedicine." *Science* 196:129–36.

Ergil, K. 1996. "China's Traditional Medicine." In *Fundamentals of Complemen-*

tary and Alternative Medicine, edited by M. Micozzi, 185–230. New York: Churchill Livingstone.

Etkin, N. 1990. "Ethnopharmacology: Biological and Behavioral Perspectives in the Study of Indigenous Medicines." In *Medical Anthropology: Contemporary Theory and Method*, edited by T. Johnson and C. Sargent, 149–58. New York: Praeger.

Fagin, C. 1994. "Women and Nursing: A Historical Perspective." In *An Unfinished Revolution: Women and Health Care in America*, edited by E. Friedman, 159–76. New York: United Hospital Fund of New York.

Feagin, J., H. Vera, and B. Zsembik. 1996. "Multiculturalism: A Democratic Basis for U.S. Society." In *Perspectives on Sociology*, edited by C. Calhoun and G. Ritzer, 1–22. New York: McGraw-Hill.

Fee, E. 1989. "Henry E. Sigerist: From the Social Production of Disease to Medical Management and Scientific Socialism." *Milbank Quarterly* 67(suppl. 1):127–50.

Ferraro, G., W. Trevathan, and J. Levy. 1994. *Anthropology: An Applied Perspective*. San Francisco: West Publishing Co.

Fischoff, B., S. Lichtenstein, P. Slovic, S. L. Derby, and R. L. Keeny. 1981. *Acceptable Risk*. New York: Cambridge University Press.

Flexner, A. 1910. *Medical Education in the United States and Canada: A Report to the Carnegie Foundation for the Advancement of Teaching*, Bulletin 4. Boston: D. B. Updike, The Merrymount Press.

Flint, M. 1975. "The Menopause: Reward or Punishment?" *Psychosomatics* 16: 161–63.

Foster, G. 1976. "Disease Etiologies in Non-Western Medical Systems." *American Anthropologist* 78:773–82.

Foster, G. 1978. "Medical Anthropology: Some Contrasts with Medical Sociology." In *Health and the Human Condition: Perspectives on Medical Anthropology*, edited by M. Logan and E. Hunt Jr., 2–11. North Scituate, MA: Duxbury Press.

Foster, G. 1994. *Hippocrates' Latin American Legacy: Humoral Medicine in the New World*. Amsterdam: Gordon and Breach.

Foucault, M. 1975 [1963]. *The Birth of the Clinic*. New York: Vintage.

Fox, R. 1977. "The Medicalization and Demedicalization of American Society." *Daedalus* 106(9):9–22.

———. 1989. *The Sociology of Medicine: A Participant Observer's View*. Englewood Cliffs, NJ: Prentice-Hall.

———. 1994. "The Entry of U.S. Bioethics into the 1990s." In *A Matter of Principles?: Ferment in U.S. Bioethics*, edited by E. DuBose, R. Hamel, and L. O'Connell, 21–71. Valley Forge, PA: Trinity Press International.

Frankenberg, R. 1994. "The Impact of HIV/AIDS on Concepts Relating to Risk and Culture Within British Community Epidemiology: Candidates or Targets for Prevention." *Social Science and Medicine* 18(10):1325–35.

Fraser, S., ed. 1995. *The Bell Curve Wars: Race, Intelligence, and the Future of America*. New York: Basic Books.

Frazer, J. 1942 [1922]. *The Golden Bough: A Study in Magic and Religion*, abridged ed. New York: The Macmillan Co.

Frazier, H., and F. Mosteller, eds. 1995. *Medicine Worth Paying For*. Cambridge, MA.: Harvard University Press.

Freeman, H., R. Blendon, L. Aiken, S. Sudman, C. Mullinix, and C. Corey. 1990. "Americans Report on Their Access to Health Care." In *The Nation's Health*, edited by P. Lee and C. Estes, 309–19. 3rd ed. Boston: Jones and Bartlett.

Freidson, E. 1960. "Client Control and Medical Practice." *American Journal of Sociology* 65:374–82.

———. 1970. *Profession of Medicine: A Study of the Sociology of Applied Knowledge*. New York: Harper and Row.

Freund, P., and M. McGuire. 1995. *Health, Illness, and the Social Body: A Critical Sociology*. 2nd ed. Englewood Cliffs, NJ: Prentice-Hall.

Friedman, E. 1994. "Women and Health Care: The Bramble and the Rose." In *An Unfinished Revolution: Women and Health Care in America*, edited by E. Friedman, 1–12. New York: United Hospital Fund of New York.

Fuller, J., and P. Toon. 1988. *Medical Practice in a Multicultural Society*. London: Heinemann.

Funkhouser, S., and D. Moser. 1990. "Is Health Care Racist?" *Advanced Nursing Science* 12(2):47–55.

Furnham, A., and R. Beard. 1995. "Health, Just World Beliefs and Coping Style Preferences in Patients of Complementary and Orthodox Medicine." *Social Science and Medicine* 40(10):1425–32.

Galanti, G. 1991. *Caring for Patients from Different Cultures: Case Studies from American Hospitals*. Philadelphia: University of Pennsylvania Press.

Gallagher, E., and J. Subedi. 1995. *Global Perspectives on Health Care*. Englewood Cliffs, NJ: Prentice-Hall.

Garrett, L. 1994. *The Coming Plague*. New York: Farrar, Straus and Giroux.

Gatter, P. 1995. "Anthropology, HIV and Contingent Identities." *Social Science and Medicine* 41(11):1523–33.

Gayford, J. 1994. "Domestic Violence." In *Violence in Health Care: A Practical Guide to Coping with Violence and Caring for Victims*, edited J. Shepherd, 117–34. New York: Oxford University Press.

Gerhardt, U. 1989. *Ideas about Illness*. New York: New York University Press.

Gerth, H., and C. Mills, eds. 1958. *From Max Weber: Essays in Sociology*. New York: Galaxy.

Gesler, W. 1991. *The Cultural Geography of Health Care*. Pittsburgh: University of Pittsburgh Press.

Ginzberg, E. 1990. *The Medical Triangle: Physicians, Politicians, and the Public*. Cambridge, MA: Harvard University Press.

Glass, R. 1996. "The Patient-Physician Relationship: JAMA Focuses on the Center of Medicine." *Journal of the American Medical Association* 275(2):147–48.

Glazer, N. 1994. "Multiculturalism and Public Policy." In *Values and Public Policy*, edited by H. Aaron, T. Mann, and T. Taylor, 113–45. Washington, DC: The Brookings Institution.

Goffman, E. 1959. *The Presentation of Self in Everyday Life*. New York: Doubleday.

Good, B. 1994. *Medicine, Rationality, and Experience: An Anthropological Perspective.* Cambridge: Cambridge University Press.

Good, B., and M. Delvecchio Good. 1993. " 'Learning Medicine': The Constructing of Medical Knowledge at Harvard Medical School." In *Knowledge, Power and Practice*, edited by S. Lindenbaum and M. Lock, 81–107. Los Angeles: University of California Press.

Gordon, D. 1991. "Female Circumcision and Genital Operations in Egypt and the Sudan: A Dilemma for Medical Anthropology." *Medical Anthropology Quarterly* 5(1):3–14.

Gordon, G. 1966. *Role Theory and Illness.* New Haven: College and University Press.

Gregor, T. 1985. *Anxious Pleasures.* Chicago: University of Chicago Press.

Groce, N., and I. Zola. 1993. "Multiculturalism, Chronic Illness, and Disability." *Pediatrics* 91(5):1048–55.

Gross, D. 1992. *Discovering Anthropology.* Mountain View, CA: Mayfield Publishing Co.

Grossman, Richard. 1985. *The Other Medicines.* New York: Doubleday & Co., Inc.

Gustafson, J. 1990. "Moral Discourse About Medicine: A Variety of Forms." *Journal of Medicine and Philosophy* 15:125–42.

Hahn, R. 1984. "Rethinking 'Illness' and 'Disease'." *Contributions to Asian Studies* 18:1–23.

———. 1995. *Sickness and Healing: An Anthropological Perspective.* New Haven: Yale University Press.

Hall, E. 1980 [1959]. *The Silent Language.* Westport, CT: Greenwood Press.

Hallowell, A. 1977 [1941]. "The Social Function of Anxiety in a Primitive Society." In *Culture, Disease, and Healing: Studies in Medical Anthropology*, edited by D. Landy, 132–38. New York: Macmillan Publishing.

Hansen, W., G. Hahn, and B. Wolkenstein. 1990. "Perceived Personal Immunity: Beliefs About Susceptibility to AIDS." *Journal of Sex Research* 27(4):622–28.

Hays, R., L. McKusick, L. Pollack, R. Hillard, C. Hoff, and T. Coates. 1993. "Disclosing HIV Seropositivity to Significant Others." *AIDS* 7(3):425–31.

Hechinger, F. 1992. "Adolescent Health: A Generation at Risk." *Carnegie Quarterly* 37(4):2–16.

Helman, C. 1990. *Culture, Health and Illness.* 2nd ed. Oxford, England: Butterworth-Heinemann.

———. 1995. *Culture, Health and Illness.* 3rd ed. London: Butterworth-Heinemann.

Herek, G., and J. Capitanio. 1994. "Conspiracies, Contagion, and Compassion: Trust and Public Reactions to AIDS." *AIDS Education and Prevention* 6(4): 365–75.

Herrell, I. 1992. Transcript of 1992 Health Care Parliament, "Ethnic Minorities and Health Care: Issues and Solutions." 6–19. Albuquerque: New Mexico Health Decisions.

Hertzman, C., J. Frank, and R. Evans. 1994. "Heterogeneities in Health Status and the Determinants of Population and Health." In *Why Are Some People Healthy and Others Not?: The Determinants of Health of Populations*, edited by R. Evans, M. Barer, and T. Marmor, 67–92. New York: Aldine de Gruyter.

Heurtin-Roberts, S., and E. Reisin. 1990. "Folk Models of Hypertension Among Black Women: Problems in Illness Management." In *Anthropology and Primary Health Care*, edited by J. Coreil and D. Mull, 222–50. Boulder, CO: Westview Press.

Hingson, R., and L. Strunin. 1992. "Monitoring Adolescents' Response to the AIDS Epidemic: Changes in Knowledge, Attitudes, Beliefs, and Behaviors." In *Adolescents and AIDS: A Generation in Jeopardy*, edited by R. DiClemente, 3–16. Newbury Park, CA: Sage.

Hollingsworth, J. 1981. "Inequality in Levels of Health in England and Wales, 1891–1971." *Journal of Health and Social Behavior* 22:268–83.

Holmes, O. 1888 [1861]. "Currents and Counter-Currents in Medical Science." In *Medical Essays, 1842–1882*. Boston: Houghton, Mifflin.

Holmes, T., and R. Rahe. 1967. "The Social Readjustment Rating Scale." *Journal of Psychosomatic Research* 11:213–18.

Holohan, A. 1977. "Diagnosis: The End of Transition." In *Medical Encounters: The Experience of Illness and Treatment*, edited by A. Davis and G. Horobin, 87–97. New York: St. Martin's Press.

Hoopes, D. 1981. "Intercultural Communication Concepts and the Psychology of Intercultural Experience." In *Multicultural Education*, edited by M. Pusch, 10–38. New York: Intercultural Press.

Hufford, D. 1992. "Folk Medicine in Contemporary America." In *Herbal and Magical Medicine: Traditional Healing Today*, edited by J. Kirkland, H. Mathews, C. Sullivan III, and K. Baldwin, 14–31. Durham, NC: Duke University Press.

———. 1994. "Folklore and Medicine." In *Putting Folklore to Use*, edited by M. Jones, 117–35. Lexington: University Press of Kentucky.

Hutchinson, J. 1993. *Delayed Diagnosis of HIV/AIDS Among Women in the United States: Its Causes and Health Repercussions* (Ms. in files of the author).

Ijsselmuiden, C., and R. Faden. 1992. "Research and Informed Consent in Africa—Another Look." *New England Journal of Medicine* 326 (March 19):830–34.

Illich, I. 1976. *Medical Nemesis: The Expropriation of Health*. New York: Pantheon.

JAMA. 1993. "Update: Acquired Immunodeficiency Syndrome—United States, 1992." *Journal of the American Medical Association* 270(8):930–31.

———. 1996. *Letters to the Editor* 275(2):107–10.

Janzen, J. M. 1978. *The Quest for Therapy: Medical Pluralism in Lower Zaire*. Los Angeles: University of California Press.

Johnsen, D. 1987. "A New Threat to Pregnant Women's Autonomy." *The Hastings Center Report* 17 (August/September):33–40.

Johnson, A. 1996. *Science, Technology and Medicine. Human Arrangements: An Introduction to Sociology*. 4th ed. Dubuque, IA: Brown and Benchmark.

Johnson, M. 1987. *The Body in the Mind*. Chicago: University of Chicago Press.

Jones, J. 1992. "The Tuskegee Legacy: AIDS and the Black Community." *Hastings Center Report* 22(6):38–40.

Jordan, B. 1993. *Birth in Four Cultures: A Crosscultural Investigation of Childbirth in Yucatan, Holland, Sweden, and the United States*. 4th ed., rev. and expanded by Robbie Davis-Floyd. Prospect Heights, IL: Waveland Press.

Kalish, R., and D. Reynolds. 1981. *Death and Ethnicity: A Psychocultural Study*. Farmingdale, NY: Baywood.

Kammerer, C., and P. Symonds. 1992. "Hill Tribes Endangered at Thailand's Periphery." *Cultural Survival Quarterly* 16(3):23–25.

Kaptchuk, T. 1996. "Historical Context of the Concept of Vitalism in Complementary and Alternative Medicine." In *Fundamentals of Complementary and Alternative Medicine*, edited by M. Micozzi, 35–48. New York: Churchill Livingstone.

Kart, C. 1990. *The Realities of Aging: An Introduction to Gerontology*. 3rd ed. Boston: Allyn and Bacon.

Katchadourian, H. 1978. "Medical Perspectives on Adulthood." In *Adulthood*, edited by E. Erikson, 33–60. New York: W. W. Norton.

Kaufert, P. 1986. "Menstruation and Menstrual Change: Women in Midlife." In *Culture, Society, and Menstruation*, edited by V. Olesen and N. F. Woods, 63–76. New York: Hemisphere.

Kaufman, S. 1993. *The Healer's Tale*. Madison: University of Wisconsin Press.

Kavanagh, K., and P. Kennedy. 1992. *Promoting Cultural Diversity Strategies for Health Care Professionals*. Newbury Park, CA: Sage.

Kaw, E. 1993. "Medicalization of Racial Features: Asian American Women and Cosmetic Surgery." *Medical Anthropology Quarterly* 7(1):74–89.

Kegeles, S., N. Adler, and C. Irwin. 1988. "Sexually Active Adolescents and Condoms: Changes Over One Year in Knowledge, Attitudes and Use." *American Journal of Public Health* 78:460–67.

Kinsey, K. 1994. " 'But I Know My Man': HIV/AIDS Risk Appraisals and Heuristical Reasoning Patterns Among Childbearing Women." *Holistic Nurse Practitioner* 8(2):79–88.

Kinsey, A., W. Pomeroy, and C. Martin. 1948. *Sexual Behavior in the Human Male*. Philadelphia: W. B. Saunders.

———. 1953. *Sexual Behavior in the Human Female*. Philadelphia: W. B. Saunders.

Kleinman, A. 1984. "Indigenous Systems of Healing: Questions for Professional, Popular, and Folk Care." In *Alternative Medicines: Popular and Policy Perspectives*, edited by J. Salmon. New York: Tavistock.

———. 1986a [1978]. "Concepts and a Model for the Comparison of Medical Systems as Cultural Systems." In *Concepts of Health, Illness and Disease: A Comparative Perspective*, edited by C. Currer and M. Stacey, 29–47. Oxford: Berg Publishers.

———. 1986b. *Social Origins of Distress and Disease*. New Haven: Yale University Press.

Kleinman, J., and J. Madans. 1985. "The Effects of Maternal Smoking, Physical Stature, and Educational Attainment on the Incidence of Low Birth Weight." *American Journal of Epidemiology* 121(6):832–55.

Korbin, J. 1987. "Child Abuse and Neglect: The Cultural Context." In *The Battered Child*, edited by R. Helfer and R. Kempe, 23–41. 4th ed. Chicago: University of Chicago Press.

Korbin, J., and M. Johnston. 1982. "Steps Toward Resolving Cultural Conflict in a Pediatric Hospital." *Clinical Pediatrics* 21(5):259–63.

Kornblum, W., and J. Julian. 1995. *Social Problems*. 8th ed. Englewood Cliffs, NJ: Prentice-Hall.

Krause, E. 1977. *Power and Illness: The Political Sociology of Health and Medical Care*. New York: Elsevier.

Kreps, G., and E. Kunimoto. 1994. *Effective Communication in Multicultural Health Settings*. Thousand Oaks, CA: Sage.

Krieger, D. 1984. "Therapeutic Touch and the Metaphysics of Nursing." In *Mind, Body and Health: Toward an Integral Medicine*, edited by J. Gordon, D. Jaffe, and D. Bresler, 107–16. New York: Human Sciences Press.

Kunitz, S. 1983. *Disease Change and the Role of Medicine: The Navajo Experience*. Berkeley: University of California Press.

———. 1994. *Disease and Social Diversity: The European Impact on the Health of Non-Europeans*. New York: Oxford University Press.

Kurth, A., and M. Hutchison. 1989. "A Context for HIV Testing in Pregnancy." *Journal of Nurse-Midwifery* 34(5):259–65.

LaFleur, W. 1992. *Liquid Life: Abortion and Buddhism in Japan*. Princeton, NJ: Princeton University Press.

Laguerre, M. 1987. *Afro-Caribbean Folk Medicine*. South Hadley, MA: Bergin & Garvey.

Laine, C., and F. Davidoff. 1996. "Patient-Centered Medicine: A Professional Evolution." *Journal of the American Medical Association* 275(2):152–56.

Lakoff, G. 1987. *Women, Fire, and Dangerous Things*. Chicago: University of Chicago Press.

Landy, D., ed. 1977. *Culture, Disease, and Healing: Studies in Medical Anthropology*. New York: Macmillan Publishing.

Laqueur, T. 1990. *Making Sex: Body and Gender from the Greeks to Freud*. Cambridge, MA: Harvard University Press.

Lazarus, E. 1990. "Falling Through the Cracks: Contradictions and Barriers to Care in a Prenatal Clinic." *Medical Anthropology* 12:269–87.

Leininger, M. 1985. "Transcultural Caring: A Different Way to Help People." In *Handbook of Cross-Cultural Counseling and Therapy*, edited by P. Pedersen, 107–16. Westport, CT: Greenwood.

———. 1993. "Assumptive Premises of the Theory." In *Cultural Care Diversity and Universality Theory*, edited by M. Leininger and C. Reynolds, 15–30. Newbury Park, CA: Sage.

Leslie, C. 1976. "Introduction." In *Asian Medical Systems: A Comparative Study*, edited by C. Leslie, 1–12. Los Angeles: University of California Press.

Lester, C., and L. Saxxon. 1988. "AIDS in the Black Community: The Plague, the Politics, the People." *Death Studies* 12:563–71.

Levine, C., and N. Dubler. 1990. "Uncertain Risks and Bitter Realities: The Reproductive Choices of HIV-Infected Women." *The Milbank Quarterly* 68(3): 321–51.

Levine, L. 1997. *The Opening of the American Mind: Canons, Culture and History*. New York: Farrar, Straus and Giroux.

Lewis, D., and J. Watters. 1989. "Human Immunodeficiency Virus Seroprevalence in Female Intravenous Drug Users: The Puzzle of Black Women's Risk." *Social Science and Medicine* 29(9):1071–76.

Lewis, G. 1986. "Concepts of Health and Illness in a Sepik Society." In *Concepts of Health, Illness and Disease: A Comparative Perspective*, edited by C. Currer and M. Stacey, 119–35. Oxford, England: Berg.

Lieberman, J. 1970. *The Tyranny of the Experts: How Professionals Are Closing the Open Society*. New York: Walker and Co.

Liebow, E. 1967. *Tally's Corner: A Study of Negro Streetcorner Men*. Boston: Little Brown and Co.

Limandri, B. 1989. "Disclosure of Stigmatizing Conditions: The Discloser's Perspective." *Archives of Psychiatric Nursing* 3(2):69–78.

Lindsay, M., H. Peterson, T. Feng, et al. 1989. "Routine Antepartum Human Immunodefiency Virus Infection Screening in an Inner-City Population." *Obstetrics and Gynecology* 74(3):289–94.

Lock, M. 1988. "Introduction." In *Biomedicine Examined*, edited by M. Lock and D. Gordon, 3–16. Dordrecht, The Netherlands: Academic Publishers.

———. 1993. "The Politics of Mid-Life and Menopause." In *Knowledge, Power, and Practice: The Anthropology of Medicine and Everyday Life*, edited by S. Lindenbaum and M. Lock, 330–63. Berkeley: University of California Press.

Locke, D. 1992. *Increasing Multicultural Understanding: A Comprehensive Model*. Newbury Park, CA: Sage.

Logan, M. 1977. "Humoral Medicine in Guatemala and Peasant Acceptance of Modern Medicine." In *Culture, Disease, and Healing: Studies in Medical Anthropology*, edited by D. Landy, 487–95. New York: Macmillan Publishing.

Loustaunau, M. 1990. "Folk Medicine in the Mesilla Valley." *The World and I* 5(2):654–65.

Lowenberg, J. 1989. *Caring and Responsibility*. Philadelphia: University of Pennsylvania Press.

Luecke, R. 1993. "A New Dawn with Fingers to the World." In *A New Dawn in Guatemala: Toward a Worldwide Health Vision*, edited by R. Luecke, ix–x. Prospect Heights, IL: Waveland Press.

Lupton, D. 1994. *Medicine as Culture: Illness, Disease and the Body in Western Societies*. London: Sage.

Lyng, S. 1990. *Holistic Health and Biomedical Medicine*. New York: State University of New York Press.

Macintyre, S., and D. Oldman. 1977. "Coping with Migraine." In *Medical Encounters: The Experience of Illness and Treatment*, edited by A. Davis and G. Horobin, 55–71. New York: St. Martin's Press.

Mack, T., and R. Ross. 1989. "Risks and Benefits of Long-Term Treatment with Estrogens." *Schweizensche Medizinische Wochenschrift* 119:1811–20.

Magner, L. 1992. *A History of Medicine*. New York: Marcel Dekker.

Majumdar, B. 1995. *Culture and Health: Culture-Sensitive Training Manual for the Health Care Provider*. 4th ed. Hamilton, Ontario: McMaster University.

Manio, E., and R. Hall. 1987. "Asian Family Traditions and their Influence in Transcultural Health Care Delivery." *Children's Health Care* 15:172–77.

Marmot, M., M. Shipley, and G. Rose. 1984. "Inequalities in Death—Specific Explanations of a General Pattern." *Lancet* 83:1003–1006.

Martin, E. 1987. *The Woman in the Body: A Cultural Analysis of Reproduction.* Boston: Beacon Press.

———. 1990. "Toward an Anthropology of Immunology: The Body as Nation State." *Medical Anthropology Quarterly* 4(4):410–26.

———. 1994. *Flexible Bodies: Tracking Immunity in American Culture From the Days of Polio to the Age of AIDS.* Boston: Beacon Press.

Masters, W., and V. Johnson. 1966. *Human Sexual Response.* Boston: Little, Brown.

Mays, V., and S. Cochran. 1987. "Acquired Immunodeficiency Syndrome and Black Americans: Special Psychosocial Issues." *Public Health Reports* 102(2):224–31.

McCormick, R. 1994. "Beyond Principlism is Not Enough." In *A Matter of Principles?: Ferment in U.S. Bioethics,* edited by E. DuBose, R. Hamel, and L. O'Connell, 344–61. Valley Forge, PA: Trinity Press International.

McKnight, J. 1993. "Taking Charge of Health in a Chicago Neighborhood." In *A New Dawn in Guatemala: Toward a Worldwide Health Vision,* edited by R. Luecke, 219–27. Prospect Heights, IL: Waveland Press.

McQuillan, G., M. Khare, T. Ezzati-Rice, J. Karon, C. Schable, and R. Murphy. 1994. "The Seroepidemiology of Human Immunodeficiency Virus in the United States Household Population: NHANES III, 1988–1991." *Journal of Acquired Immune Deficiency Syndrome* 7(11):1195–1201.

Mead, M. 1935. *Sex and Temperament in Three Primitive Societies.* New York: William Morrow.

———. 1963 [1928]. *Coming of Age in Samoa: A Study of Adolescence and Sex in Primitive Society.* New York: Mentor Books.

Mechanic, D. 1962. "The Concept of Illness Behavior." *Journal of Chronic Diseases* 15:189–94.

———. 1978. *Medical Sociology.* 2nd ed. New York: The Free Press.

Meigs, A. 1983. *Food, Sex, and Pollution: A New Guinea Religion.* New Brunswick, NJ: Rutgers University Press.

The Merck Manual, 14th ed. 1982. Berkow, R., ed. Rahway, NJ: Merck Sharp & Dohme Research Laboratories.

Messina, S. 1992. *Lesbian, Gay and Bisexual Youth: At Risk and Underserved.* Washington DC: Center for Population Options.

Micozzi, M. 1996a. "Characteristics of Complementary and Alternative Medicine Systems." In *Fundamentals of Complementary and Alternative Medicine,* edited by M. Micozzi, 3–8. New York: Churchill Livingstone.

———. 1996b. *Fundamentals of Complementary and Alternative Medicine.* New York: Churchill Livingston.

Money, J. 1980. *Love and Love Sickness: The Science of Sex, Gender Difference, and Pair-bonding.* Baltimore: Johns Hopkins University Press.

Montagu, A. 1969. Letters to editor. *New York Times* (July 13): iv–13.

Monthly Forum on Women in Higher Education. 1995. 1(3):6–7.

Moore, L., P. Van Arsdale, J. Glittenberg, and R. Aldrich. 1987 [1980]. *The Biocultural Basis of Health: Expanding Views of Medical Anthropology.* Prospect Heights, IL: Waveland Press.

Morgan, L. 1989. "When Does Life Begin? A Cross-Cultural Perspective on the Personhood of Fetuses and Young Children." In *Abortion Rights and Fetal "Personhood,"* edited by E. Doerr and J. Prescott, 97–114. Long Beach, CA: Centerline Press.

Morley, P. 1978. "Culture and the Cognitive World of Traditional Medical Beliefs: Some Preliminary Considerations." In *Culture and Curing: Anthropological Perspectives on Traditional Medical Beliefs and Practices,* edited by P. Morley and R. Wallis, 1–18. Pittsburgh: University of Pittsburgh Press.

Muller, J., and B. Koenig. 1988. "On the Boundary of Life and Death: The Definition of Dying by Medical Residents." In *Biomedicine Examined,* edited by M. Lock and D. Gordon, 351–74. Dordrecht, The Netherlands: Kluwer Academic Publishers.

Mumford, E. 1983. *Medical Sociology: Patients, Providers, and Policies.* New York: Random House.

Munson, R., with C. Hoffman. 1996. *Intervention and Reflection: Basic Issues in Medical Ethics.* 5th ed. Belmont, CA: Wadsworth.

Myrdal, G. 1944. *An American Dilemma: The Negro Problem and Modern Democracy.* New York: Harper.

Naisbitt, J., and P. Aburdene. 1990. *Megatrends 2000: Ten New Directions for the 1990's.* New York: William Morrow.

Navarro, V. 1976. *Medicine Under Capitalism.* New York: Prodist.

———. 1994. "Race or Class versus Race and Class: Mortality Differentials in the United States." In *Issues in Medical Sociology,* edited by H. Schwartz, 491–504. 3rd ed. New York: McGraw-Hill.

NCHS [National Center for Health Statistics]. 1988. *Health, United States, 1987.* Washington, DC: U.S. Government Printing Office.

———. 1991. *Disability and Health: Characteristics of Persons by Limitation of Activity and Assessed Health Status, United States, 1984–88.* Advance Data, No. 197.

Ngin, C. 1985. "Indigenous Fertility Regulating Methods Among Two Chinese Communities in Malaysia." In *Women's Medicine: A Cross-Cultural Study of Indigenous Fertility Regulation,* edited by L. Newman, 25–41. New Brunswick, NJ: Rutgers University Press.

Nichols, M. 1990. "Women and Acquired Immunodeficiency Syndrome: Issues for Prevention." In *Aids and Sex: An Integrated Biomedical and Biobehavioral Approach,* edited by B. Voeller, J. Reinisch, and M. Gottlieb, 375–92. New York: Oxford University Press.

Nichter, M., and M. Nichter. 1987. "Cultural Notions of Fertility in South Asia and Their Impact on Sri Lankan Family Planning Practices." *Human Organization* 46(1):18–28.

Novak, D., G. Volk, D. Drossman, and M. Lipkin. 1993. "Medical Interviewing and Interpersonal Skills Teaching in U.S. Medical Schools." *Journal of the American Medical Association* 269:2102–5.

Nunley, M. 1995. "The Bell Curve: Too Smooth to be True." *American Behavioral Scientist* 39(1):74–83.

Nyamathi, A., P. Shuler, and M. Porche. 1990. "AIDS Educational Program for Minority Women at Risk." *Family and Community Health* 13(2):54–64.

Oliver, W. 1989. "Sexual Conquest and Patterns of Black-on-Black Violence: A Structural-Cultural Perspective." *Violence and Victims* 4(4):257–73.

Pappas, G., S. Queen, W. Hadden, and G. Fisher. 1993. "The Increasing Disparity in Mortality Between Socioeconomic Groups in the United States, 1960 and 1986." *New England Journal of Medicine* 329(July 8):103–9.

Parsons, T. 1951. *The Social System*. Glencoe, IL: Free Press.

Payer, L. 1989. *Medicine and Culture*. New York: Penguin Books.

Pelto, P., and G. Pelto. 1990. "Field Methods in Medical Anthropology." In *Medical Anthropology: Contemporary Theory and Method*, edited by T. Johnson and C. Sargent, 269–97. New York: Praeger.

Pfifferling, J. 1981. "A Cultural Prescription for Medicocentrism." In *The Relevance of Social Science for Medicine*, edited by L. Eisenberg and A. Kleinman, 197–222.

Pickin, C., and S. St. Leger. 1993. *Assessing Health Need Using the Life Cycle Framework*. Buckingham, England: Open University Press.

Pierret, J. 1995 [1983]. "The Social Meanings of Health: Paris, the Essone and the Herault." In *The Meaning of Illness: Anthropology, History and Sociology*, edited by M. Augé and C. Herzlich, 151–73. Translated from the French by K. Durnin, C. Lambein, K. Leclercq-Jones, B. Garnier, and R. Williams. London: Harwood Academic Publishers.

Pivnick, A. 1993. "HIV Infection and the Meaning of Condoms." *Culture, Medicine, and Psychiatry* 17(4):431–53.

Polednak, A. 1989. *Racial and Ethnic Differences in Disease*. New York: Oxford University Press.

Pratt, L. 1976. *Family Structure and Effective Health Behavior: The Energized Family*. Boston: Houghton Mifflin.

Prohaska, T., G. Albrecht, and J. Levy. 1990. "Determinants of Self-Perceived Risk for AIDS." *Journal of Health and Social Behavior* 31:384–94.

Quill, T. 1983. "Partnerships in Patient Care: A Contractual Approach." *Annals of Internal Medicine* 98:228–34.

Quimby, E. 1992. "Anthropological Witnessing for African-Americans: Power, Responsibility, and Choice in the Age of AIDS." In *The Time of AIDS: Social Analysis, Theory, and Method*, edited by G. Herdt and S. Lindenbaum, 159–84. Newbury Park, CA: Sage.

Reid, I. 1989. *Social Class Differences in Britain*. 3rd ed. Glasgow, Scotland: Fontana Press.

Rensberger, B. 1993, August 9–15. "Teenage Girls Are on the 'Leading Edge' of the AIDS Scourge." In *Washington Post National Weekly Edition*, 34.

Rice, D. 1990. "The Medical Care System: Past Trends and Future Projections." In *The Nation's Health*, edited by P. Lee and C. Estes, 72–93. 3rd ed. Boston: Jones and Bartlett.

Richardson, L. 1988. *The Dynamics of Sex and Gender: A Sociological Perspective*. New York: Harper and Row.

Rivera, G., Jr. 1990. "AIDS and Mexican Folk Medicine." *Sociology and Social Research* 75(1):3–7.

Robertson, L., and M. Heagarty. 1975. *Medical Sociology: A General Systems Approach*. Chicago: Nelson-Hall Publishers.

Romalis, S., ed. 1981. *Childbirth: Alternatives to Medical Control*. Austin: University of Texas Press.

Romanucci-Ross, L. 1977 [1969]. "The Hierarchy of Resort in Curative Practices: The Admiralty Islands, Melanesia." In *Culture, Disease, and Healing: Studies in Medical Anthropology*, edited by D. Landy, 481–87. New York: Macmillan Publishing.

Rosen, G. 1974. *From Medical Police to Social Medicine: Essays on the History of Health Care*. New York: Science History Publications.

Rosenstock, I. 1966. "Why People Use Health Services." *Milbank Memorial Fund Quarterly* 44:94–127.

Rothman, B. 1994. "Midwives in Transition: The Structure of a Clinical Revolution." In *Dominant Issues in Medical Sociology*, edited by H. Schwartz, 104–12. 3rd ed. New York: McGraw-Hill.

Sacks, K. 1974. "Engels Revisited: Women, the Organization of Production, and Private Property." In *Women, Culture, and Society*, edited by M. Rosaldo and L. Lamphere, 207–22. Stanford, CA: Stanford University Press.

Salmon, J., ed. 1984. *Alternative Medicines: Popular and Policy Perspectives*. New York: Tavistock Publications.

Schlegel, A., and H. Barry III. 1991. *Adolescence: An Anthropological Inquiry*. New York: Free Press.

Schlesinger, A., Jr. 1992. *The Disuniting of America*. New York: W. W. Norton and Co.

Schmidt, D. 1978. "The Family as the Unit of Medical Care." *Journal of Family Practice* 7(2):303–13.

Schoenborn, C., S. Marsh, and A. Hardy. 1994. "AIDS Knowledge and Attitudes for 1992: Data From the National Health Interview Survey." In *Advance Data From Vital and Health Statistics, No. 243*. Hyattsville, MD: National Center for Health Statistics.

Schweitzer, M. 1983. "The Elders: Cultural Dimensions of Aging in Two American Indian Communities." In *Growing Old in Different Societies*, edited by J. Sokolovsky, 168–78. Belmont, CA: Wadsworth.

Scully, D., and P. Bart. 1979. "A Funny Thing Happened on the Way to the Orifice: Women in Gynecology Textbooks." In *The Cultural Crisis of Modern Medicine*, edited by J. Ehrenreich, 212–26. New York: Monthly Review Press.

Shedlin, M. 1982. "Anthropology and Family Planning: Culturally Appropriate Intervention in a Mexican Community." Ph.D. dissertation. Columbia University.

Shorter, E. 1985. *Bedside Manners*. New York: Simon and Schuster.

Shryock, R. 1966. "The American Physician in 1846 and in 1946: A Study in Professional Contrasts." In *Medicine in America: Historical Essays*, edited by R. Shryock, 149–76. Baltimore: Johns Hopkins Press.

Shweder, R. 1991. *Thinking Through Cultures: Expeditions in Cultural Psychology*. Cambridge, MA: Harvard University Press.

Sigerist, H. 1960 [1947]. "Medical History in the United States: Past-Future." In *On the History of Medicine*, edited by F. Marti-Ibanez, 233–50. New York: MD Publications.

Singer, M. 1995. "Beyond the Ivory Tower: Critical Praxis in Medical Anthropology." *Medical Anthropology Quarterly* 9(1):80–106.

Singer, M., F. Valentin, H. Baer, and Z. Jia. 1992. "Why Does Juan Garcia Have a Drinking Problem? The Perspective of Critical Medical Anthropology." *Medical Anthropology* 14(1):77–108.

Slater, V. 1996. "Healing Touch." In *Fundamentals of Complementary and Alternative Medicine*, edited by M. Micozzi, 121–36. New York: Churchill Livingstone.

Snow, L. 1993. *Walkin' Over Medicine*. Boulder, CO: Westview Press.

Snow, L., and S. Johnson. 1978. "Folklore, Food, Female Reproductive Cycle." *Ecology of Food and Nutrition* 7:41–49.

Sobo, E. 1992. " 'Unclean Deeds': Menstrual Taboos and Binding 'Ties' in Rural Jamaica." In *Anthropological Approaches to the Study of Ethnomedicine*, edited by M. Nichter, 101–26. New York: Gordon and Breach.

———. 1993. *One Blood: The Jamaican Body*. Albany: State University of New York Press.

———. 1994. "The Sweetness of Fat: Health, Procreation, and Sociability in Rural Jamaica." In *Body Image and Social Meaning*, edited by N. Sault, 132–54. New Brunswick, NJ: Rutgers University Press.

———. 1995. *Choosing Unsafe Sex: AIDS-Risk Denial among Disadvantaged Women*. Philadelphia: University of Pennsylvania Press.

———. 1996a. "Abortion Traditions in Rural Jamaica." *Social Science and Medicine* 42(4):495–508.

———. 1996b. "The Jamaican Body's Role in Emotional Experience and Sense Perception." *Culture, Medicine and Psychiatry* 20:313–42.

———. 1997. "Self-disclosure and Self-construction among HIV-Positive People: The Rhetorical Uses of Stereotypes and Sex." *Anthropology and Medicine* 4(1):67–87.

Sokol, E. 1992. "A Formula for Disaster." *Multinational Monitor* (March):9–13.

Soroka, M., and G. Bryjac. 1995. *Social Problems: A World at Risk*. Boston: Allyn and Bacon.

Stack, C. 1974. *All Our Kin: Strategies for Survival in a Black Community*. New York: Harper and Row.

Stafford, A. 1978. "The Application of Clinical Anthropology to Medical Practice: Case Study of Recurrent Abdominal Pain in a Preadolescent Mexican-American Female." In *The Anthropology of Health*, edited by E. Bauwens, 12–22. St. Louis: C. V. Mosby.

Stanford, D. 1977. "All About Sex . . . After Middle Age." *American Journal of Nursing* 77(4):608–11.

Starr, P. 1982. *The Social Transformation of American Medicine*. New York: Basic Books.

Stine, G. 1993. *Acquired Immune Deficiency Syndrome: Biological, Medical, Social, and Legal Issues*. Englewood Cliffs, NJ: Prentice-Hall.

Suchman, E. 1965. "Social Patterns of Illness and Medical Care." *Journal of Health and Human Behavior* 6:2–16.

Sullivan, R. 1994. "Sanguine Practices: A Historical and Historiographic Reconsideration of Heroic Therapy in the Age of Rush." *Bulletin of the History of Medicine* 68:211–34.

Syme, S., and L. Berkman. 1994. "Social Class, Susceptibility, and Sickness." In

The Sociology of Health and Illness: Critical Perspectives, edited by P. Conrad and R. Kern, 29–35. 4th ed. New York: St. Martin's.

Szasz, T., and M. Hollender. 1956. "A Contribution to the Philosophy of Medicine: The Basic Models of the Doctor-Patient Relationship." *Journal of the American Medical Association* 97:585–88.

Tanner, W., and R. Pollack. 1988. "The Effect of Condom Use and Erotic Instructions on Attitudes Toward Condoms." *Journal of Sex Research* 25(4):537–41.

Taylor, C., and D. Lourea. 1992. "HIV Prevention: A Dramaturgical Analysis and Practical Guide to Creating Safer Sex Interventions." In *Rethinking AIDS Prevention*, edited by R. Bolton and M. Singer, 105–46. New York: Gordon and Breach Science Publishers.

Taylor, J., J. Krieger, D. Reay, R. Davis, R. Harruff, and L. Cheney. 1996. "Prone Sleep Position and the Sudden Infant Death Syndrome in King County, Washington: A Case-Control Study." *Journal of Pediatrics* (Pt. 1 of 5) (May) 128:626–30.

Thompson, J., T. Yager, and J. Martin. 1993. "Estimated Condom Failure and Frequency of Condom Use Among Gay Men." *American Journal of Public Health* 83(10):1409–12.

Toubia, N. 1994. "Female Circumcision as a Public Health Issue." *New England Journal of Medicine* 331(11):712–16.

Turner, B. 1984. *The Body and Society*. Oxford: Blackwell.

———. 1995. *Medical Power and Social Knowledge*. 2nd ed. London: Sage.

Twaddle, A. 1969. "Health Decisions and Sick Role Variations: An Exploration." *Journal of Health and Social Behavior* 10:105–14.

Twaddle, A., and R. Hessler. 1987. *A Sociology of Health*. 2nd ed. New York: Macmillan.

United Nations. 1978. *International Bill of Human Rights*. New York: United Nations Office of Public Information.

U.S. Bureau of the Census. 1986. Household Wealth and Asset Ownership: 1984. *Current Population Reports*, ser. P-70, no. 7. Washington, DC: U.S. Government Printing Office.

U.S. Bureau of the Census. 1990. Household and Family Characteristics: March 1990 and 1989. *Current Population Reports*, ser. P-20, no. 447. Washington, DC: U.S. Government Printing Office.

U.S. Bureau of the Census. 1993a. Current Population Reports, Special Studies: (P23–178RV), *Sixty-Five Plus in America*, 2–9. Washington, DC: U.S. Government Printing Office.

U.S. Bureau of the Census. 1993b. *Population Projections of the United States, by Age, Sex, Race, and Hispanic Origin: 1995 to 2050*. ser. P-25, no. 1104. Washington, DC: U.S. Government Printing Office.

U.S. Bureau of the Census. 1995. Washington, DC: U.S. Government Printing Office.

U.S. Bureau of the Census. 1996. Washington, DC: U.S. Government Printing Office.

U.S. Department of Health and Human Services. 1992. *Healthy People 2000: National Health Promotion and Disease Prevention Objectives*. Boston: Jones and Bartlett.

Verbrugge, L. 1990. "Pathways of Health and Death." In *Women, Health and Medicine: A Historical Handbook*, edited by R. Apple, 41–79. New York: Garland.

Voeller, B. 1990. "Heterosexual Anal Intercourse: An AIDS Risk Factor." In *AIDS and Sex: An Integrated Biomedical and Biobehavioral Approach*, edited by B. Voeller, J. Reinisch, and M. Gottlieb, 276–311. New York: Oxford University Press.

Vogel, V. 1990. *American Indian Medicine*. Norman: University of Oklahoma Press.

Waitzkin, H. 1983. *The Second Sickness: Contradictions of Capitalist Health Care.* New York: The Free Press.

———. 1985. "Information Giving in Medical Care." *Journal of Health and Social Behavior* 26 (June):81–101.

Waldron, I. 1993. "Recent Trends in Sex Mortality Ratios for Adults in Developed Countries." *Social Science and Medicine* 36(4):451–62.

Waldron, I. 1994. "What Do We Know about Causes of Sex Differences in Mortality? A Review of the Literature." In *The Sociology of Health & Illness: Critical Perspectives*, edited by P. Conrad and R. Kern, 42–55. New York: St. Martin's Press.

Walker, A., and P. Parmar. 1993. *Warrior Marks: Female Genital Mutilation and the Sexual Blinding of Women*. New York: Harcourt Brace and Co.

Walker, R. 1991. *AIDS Today, Tomorrow: an Introduction to the HIV Epidemic in America*. Atlantic Highlands, NJ: Humanities Press International.

Ward, D. 1993. "Women and the Work of Caring." *Second Opinion* 19(2):11–25.

Ward, M. 1990. "The Politics of Adolescent Pregnancy: Turf and Teens in Louisiana." In *Births and Power: Social Change and the Politics of Reproduction*, edited by W. Handwerker, 147–64. San Francisco: Westview Press.

———. 1993a. "A Different Disease: AIDS and Health Care for Women in Poverty." *Culture, Medicine, and Psychiatry* 17(4):413–30.

———. 1993b. "Poor and Positive: Two Contrasting Views From Inside the AIDS Epidemic." *Practicing Anthropology* 15(4):59–61.

Wardwell, W. 1972. "Limited, Marginal, and Quasi-Practitioners." In *Handbook of Medical Sociology*, edited by H. Freeman, S. Levine, and L. Reeder, 250–73. Englewood Cliffs, NJ: Prentice-Hall.

Watkins, A. 1996. "Contemporary Context of Complementary and Alternative Medicine: Integrated Mind-Body Medicine." In *Fundamentals of Complementary and Alternative Medicine*, edited by M. Micozzi, 49–63. New York: Churchill Livingstone.

Wedenoja, W., and E. Sobo. 1997. "Culture and Unconscious Motivation." In *The Psychological Bases of Culture*, edited by I. Al-Issa, 159–77. New Brunswick, NJ: Rutgers University Press.

Weinberg, M., and C. Williams. 1988. "Black Sexuality: A Test of Two Theories." *Journal of Sex Research* 25(2):197–218.

Weinstein, N. 1989. "Perceptions of Personal Susceptibility to Harm." In *Primary Prevention of AIDS: Psychological Approaches*, edited by V. Mays, G. Albee, and S. Schneider, 142–67. Newbury Park, CA: Sage.

Weiss, G., and L. Lonnquist. 1994. *The Sociology of Health, Healing and Illness.* Englewood Cliffs, NJ: Prentice-Hall.

Westat, Incorporated. 1988. *Study Findings: Study of National Incidence of Child Abuse and Neglect*. Washington, DC: U.S. Department of Health and Human Services.

Whiteford, M., and J. Friedl. 1992. *The Human Portrait: Introduction to Cultural Anthropology*. 3rd ed. Englewood Cliffs, NJ: Prentice-Hall.

Whitehead, M. 1990. "The Health Divide." In *Inequalities in Health*, edited by P. Townsend and N. Davidson, 222–356. London: Penguin Books.

WHO [World Health Organization]. 1994, 4 January. *The Current Global Situation of the HIV/AIDS Pandemic–Global Programme on AIDS Report*. Geneva, Switzerland: WHO.

Widom, C. 1989. "The Cycle of Violence." *Science* 244 (April):160–66.

Williams, G., III. 1993. "Mind, Body, Spirit: The Dark Side of Hope: Seeing the Holes in the Holistic Movement." *Longevity* 28:77–78.

Williams, R., Jr. 1970. *American Society: A Sociological Interpretation*. New York: Knopf.

Wilson, R. 1966. *Feminine Forever*. New York: M. Evans and Co.

Wilson, W. 1987. *The Truly Disadvantaged*. Chicago: University of Chicago Press.

Wohl, S. 1984. *The Medical Industrial Complex*. New York: Harmony.

Wolf, N. 1991. *The Beauty Myth: How Images of Beauty Are Used Against Women*. New York: William Morrow and Co.

Worth, D. 1990. "Minority Women and AIDS: Culture, Race, and Gender." In *Cultural Aspects of AIDS*, edited by D. Feldman, 111–36. New York: Praeger Publishers.

Young, A. 1982. "The Anthropologies of Illness and Sickness." *Annual Reviews in Anthropology* 11:257–85.

———. 1983. "The Relevance of Traditional Medical Cultures to Modern Primary Health Care." *Social Science and Medicine* 17(16):1205–11.

———. 1986 [1976]. "Internalising and Externalising Medical Systems: an Ethiopian Example." In *Concepts of Health, Illness and Disease: A Comparative Perspective*, edited by C. Currer and M. Stacey, 139–60. Oxford, England: Berg Publishers.

Young, J., and L. Garro. 1982. "Choice of Treatment in Two Mexican Communities." *Social Science and Medicine* 16:1453–65.

———. *Medical Choice in a Mexican Village*, Reissue with Changes. Prospect Heights, IL: Waveland.

Zborowski, M. 1952. "Cultural Components in Response to Pain." *Journal of Social Issues* 8:16–30.

Zola, I. 1966. "Culture and Symptoms: An Analysis of Patients: Presenting Complaints." *American Sociological Review* 31:615–30.

———. 1972. "Medicine as an Institution of Social Control." *Sociological Review* 20:487–504.

———. 1983. *Socio-Medical Inquiries: Recollections, Reflections, and Reconsiderations*. Philadelphia: Temple University Press.

Index